THE ART OF
MINDFULNESS

CREATIVE ART THERAPY PRACTICES FOR THE MENTAL & EMOTIONAL WELL-BEING OF TEENS

Eme L. Williams

Book Cover by Eme L. Williams
1st edition 2024

ISBN: 979-8-9902561-0-1

To those who are suffering -
Let art be your guide on the journey to healing.

Acknowledgments

The publication of this book couldn't have happened without the unwavering and constant support of these dedicated people who I am forever thankful:

Project Advisory Team

Rose Stoloff, LCSW, Project Advisor and Upper School Counselor at The Athenian School
Sumita Bhandari, Executive Director, Discovery Counseling Center of the San Ramon Valley
Christopher Duerrmeier, LMFT, Clinical Director, Discovery Counseling Center of the San Ramon Valley
Caroline Miller, AMFT, Discovery Counseling Center of the San Ramon Valley
Dana Power, AMFT, Discovery Counseling Center of the San Ramon Valley
James Hoban, AMFT, Discovery Counseling Center of the San Ramon Valley
Dina Ramaha, LCSW, Founder, Conscious Mind Therapy Institute

Girl Scout Support

Ashley Carter, Gold Award Coordinator, Girl Scouts of Northern California
Winnie Kubik, Highest Awards Manager, Girl Scouts of Northern California
Michelle Maddaus, Girl Scout Troop 30302, Co-Leader
Karen Zaritsky, Girl Scout Troop 30302, Co-Leader

Family and Community

Mom and Dad
Kim Holmes, Educator, Danville Town Commissioner, Past President of the San Ramon Valley Historical Society Board of Directors
Robert Combs, Chair, Discovery Counseling Center of the San Ramon Valley Board of Directors

Table of Contents

Introduction

"Make sure your worst enemy doesn't live between your own two ears."

– Laird Hamilton

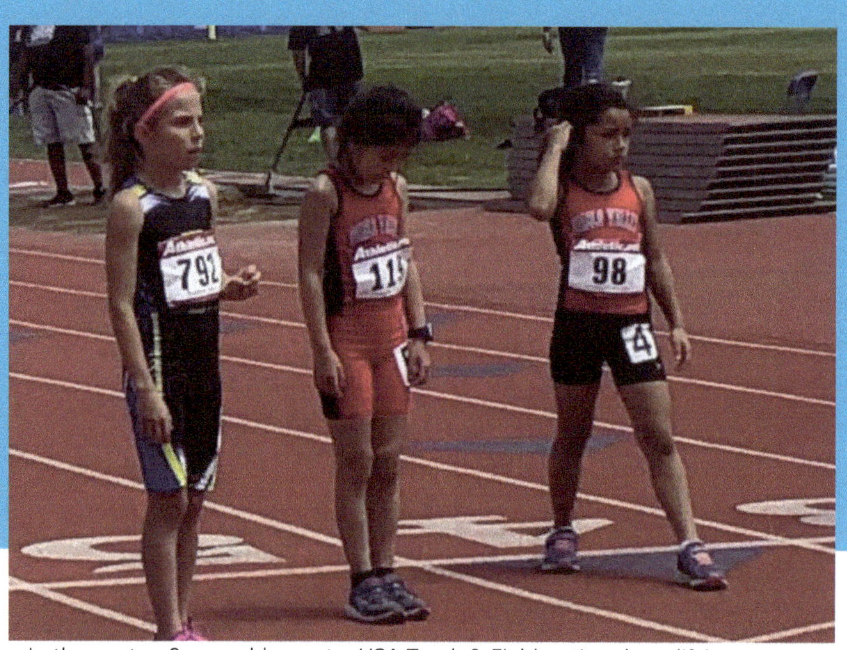

In the center: 9 year-old me at a USA Track & Field national qualifying meet, trying to manage my anxiety before the race.

Dear Reader,

Welcome to "The Art of Mindfulness" art therapy book. I'm Eme, and I'm so happy to share my mental health practices with you. Like many of you, I've faced my own challenges with performance anxiety, often struggling to find calm and clear my head in anxious moments. I've discovered a soothing escape in art, whether it was sketching in my notebook or immersing myself in a painting. It was eye-opening to see how art could be therapeutic, not just for me but for others too, especially teens going through similar struggles.

My research on this subject revealed that the issue of mental health is far more widespread and impactful in our lives than we realize or acknowledge. In 2021, U.S. Surgeon General Dr. Vivek H. Murthy issued a Mental Health Advisory describing the challenges young people face today as "uniquely hard to navigate," and called the mental health effects of these challenges "devastating." He states that "Recent national surveys of young people have shown alarming increases in the prevalence of certain mental health challenges - in 2019 one in three high school students and half of female students reported feelings of sadness or hopelessness, an overall increase of 40 percent from 2009."

Dr. Murthy's advisory is consistent with a finding in a 2019 study published by the National Academies Press, *Vibrant and Healthy Kids: Aligning Science, Practice, and Policy to Advance Health Equity*. This study notes that for children in the United States, "ailments of the past have been supplanted with chronic physical (e.g., diabetes, asthma, obesity) and socio-emotional (e.g., depression, anxiety) conditions."[1]

But there's hope. Dr. Murthy emphasizes that these mental health issues, while widespread, are both treatable and preventable. This inspired me to create this resource to help others *manage* anxiety through mindfulness practices. This book is written for teens and non-profit mental health organizations who work with them, but anyone can benefit from these exercises.

I warmly invite you to explore this book and embrace its practices of mindfulness. I hope you find these techniques helpful in managing the anxieties in your daily life. Remember, patience is key. Take your time with each activity, as this journey is uniquely yours.

Happy exploring, and I hope you find peace and healing through art.

Warm regards,

Eme

#ArtIsMyTherapy

---

[1] National Academies of Sciences, Engineering, and Medicine. 2019. Vibrant and Healthy Kids: Aligning Science, Practice, and Policy to Advance Health Equity. Washington, DC: The National Academies Press. https://doi.org/10.17226/25466.

Anxiety and Art Therapy

*"Every artist dips his brush in his own soul,
and paints his own nature into his pictures."*

– Henry Ward Beecher

What is Anxiety and Types of Anxiety Disorders

Anxiety is like that nervous feeling you get before a big test or presentation. It's a normal reaction when we face stuff that's stressful or new. But for some people, this feeling gets really intense and can make it hard for them to do everyday activities. There are different types of anxiety disorders:[2]

Generalized Anxiety Disorder (GAD): When you're constantly worried about everything, even small things.

Panic Disorder: When you have sudden attacks of intense fear that can make you feel like you're losing control.

Social Anxiety Disorder: When you're super scared of being judged or embarrassed in social situations

Specific Phobias: When you have an extreme fear of something specific, like spiders or heights.

Agoraphobia: When you're scared of places or situations that might make you panic and feel trapped or embarrassed.

Separation Anxiety Disorder: When you're really scared about being away from home or separated from people you're close to.

Selective Mutism: When kids don't talk at all in certain places like school, even though they can speak normally at home.

---

[2] www.psychology.org

Common Triggers for Anxiety

There are many different things that can trigger anxiety, including:

1. **Health Issues**: Like getting a scary health diagnosis or a lack of exercise or sleep.

2. **Medications**: Some medicines can make anxiety worse.

3. **Caffeine**: That energy drink might wake you up, but it could also ramp up your anxiety.

4. **Skipping Meals**: Not eating regularly can drop your blood sugar levels and lead to feelings of anxiety.

5. **Negative Thinking**: Worrying about past events or future ones can trigger anxiety.

6. **Financial Concerns**: Worrying about money can cause a lot of stress.

7. **Experiences with "-isms"** such as racism, sexism, or ableism.

8. **Past experiences of trauma** such as abuse, assault, being in an accident or natural disaster.

Specifically for teens, the common anxiety triggers include: [3,4]

1. **Social Situations**: Parties, meals, and other social occasions where there are lots of other people, including strangers, can cause stress or even panic.

2. **Performances or Presentations**: Situations where teens have to perform or present in front of people can be extremely strenuous.[1]

3. **Family Stress**: If your family home is a place of constant stress, this might trigger a teen's anxiety.[1]

4. **Negative Rumination**: A teen might dwell on negative moments, assume the worst outcomes and be extremely self-critical.

5. **Puberty**: Going through puberty before or after their friends is a big trigger.

6. **Academic Stress**: Stress related to schoolwork, examinations, and transitions between school years can lead to anxiety.[3]

7. **Social Media Engagement**: Greater levels of social media engagement can contribute to anxiety.

8. **Economic Stress**: Worrying about financial issues can cause a lot of stress.

---

[3] https://www.teenrehab.org/resources/helping-your-teen/common-triggers-for-teen-anxiety/

[4] https://ballardbrief.byu.edu/issue-briefs/the-rise-of-anxiety-and-depression-among-young-adults-in-the-united-states

Art Therapy and its Benefits for Anxiety

"Art washes away from the soul the dust of everyday life."
– Pablo Picasso

A question often asked is "What is art therapy and how does it work?" Art therapy is a form of psychotherapy that uses creative processes to better understand ourselves, our feelings, and to reflect and gain insights. By learning how to be more self-aware, we can explore and process difficult experiences to heal emotionally and mentally. These tools will eventually equip us with healthy coping techniques to manage our emotions more effectively.

Think of art therapy as a way to visually journal what's going on in our minds and hearts. By creating art, we can uncover and understand the root of our feelings. It's like having a visual conversation with ourselves, where we can acknowledge these emotions and start learning new ways to respond to them. It's not just about making art; it's about discovering what the art says about us and using that knowledge to grow and heal. It's been said that *"you've got to feel it to heal it."* Some things to keep in mind:

- **What is Mindfulness and how can it control anxiety?** Well, mindfulness is a skill people often use to practice paying more attention to the present moment, or being more aware of yourself and your surroundings. You can achieve mindfulness practice in a variety of ways, including mindful breathing, meditation, and even art! All of these techniques allow the individual to have more of a sense of control over their emotions.

- **Art therapy is all about expression, not perfection**. Remember, when doing art, it's not a competition and you don't need to be an artist to benefit from it. So, don't stress about your art skills – or think you don't have any. This art therapy book is here to help you, regardless of your experience with art. Just dive in and enjoy the process!

- **Experiment with different mediums and methods**. As you journey through this book, you'll get to try your hand at journaling and self-reflection, alongside experimenting with various artistic methods. Whether it's drawing, creating collages, sculpting or painting, you'll have the chance to explore and express yourself in different ways. So, get ready to dive into a world of creativity and self-discovery!

- **Use the prompts to guide self-expression**. In this art journey, you'll find yourself expressing your thoughts and feelings through art by responding to prompts. These prompts are open to your own interpretation, so feel free to express what they mean to you in your own unique way. Each art activity is an opportunity for you to explore and convey your perspective creatively.

- **Self-reflection through awareness**. After you complete an art activity, take some time to reflect on both your artwork and your feelings. Art therapy involves a lot of self-reflection, so it's important to look closely at your creation and think about the emotions it brings up. Remember, there's no right or wrong way to feel about your art. It's all about noticing how different things, like your artwork, can influence your emotions.

Some questions to consider when reflecting on your work:

1. What feelings came up as you made the artwork?
2. What do the colors mean to you?
3. What title would you give your art?
4. How does this art relate to your life right now?
5. If your art had a message, what would it say to you?

Setting Up for Self Expression

"The moods and qualities of nature and the revelations of great art are difficult to define; we can grasp them only in the depths of our perceptive spirit."

– Ansel Adams

Setting Up Your Space

Creating a Safe and Comfortable Environment

It's crucial that you find a safe and comfortable environment to practice art therapy. When you are in your safe space, it's much easier to be present and open up about how you feel in that moment without fear of judgment.

Gathering Art Supplies

Each activity will require different art supplies, but here's a general budget-friendly list of things you will need to collect prior to participating in the art therapy activities:

- Pen or pencil
- Colored pens or pencils
- Colored markers, sharpies
- Acrylic or easily washable paint
- A set of paintbrushes
- Container of water
- Extra paper
- Scissors
- Glue
- Air dry/modeling clay
- Colored construction paper
- Balloons

Using The Psychology of Colors to Express Emotions

Fun fact, the colors that you see and experience can affect how you feel. Warm-toned colors, such as red, orange, and yellow typically represent sunlight and warmth to stimulate energy and excitement. On the other hand, cool-toned colors, such as blue, indigo, and violet evoke a sense of calm and relaxation. Artists tend to use cooler hues for less stimulating, soothing art pieces.

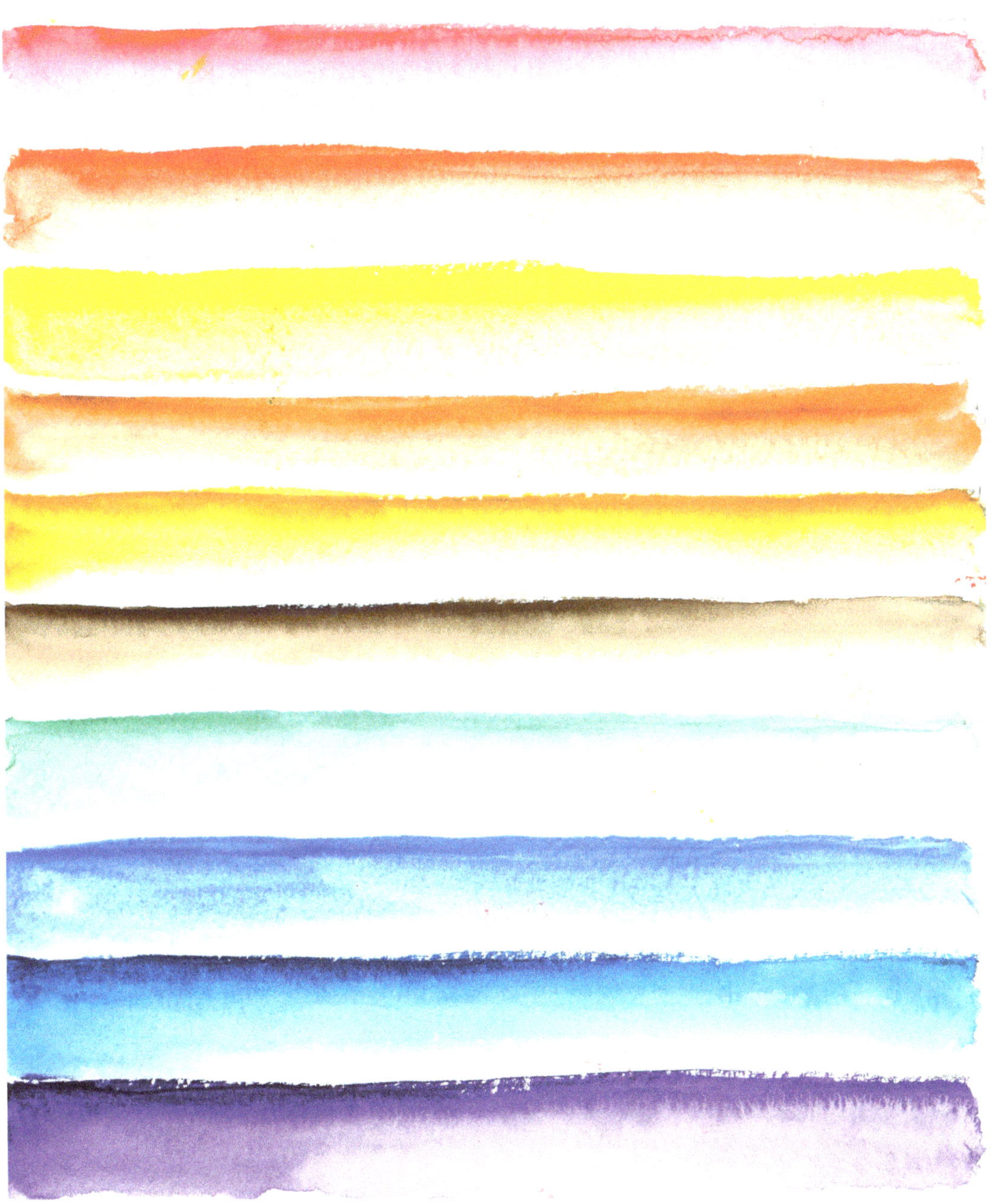

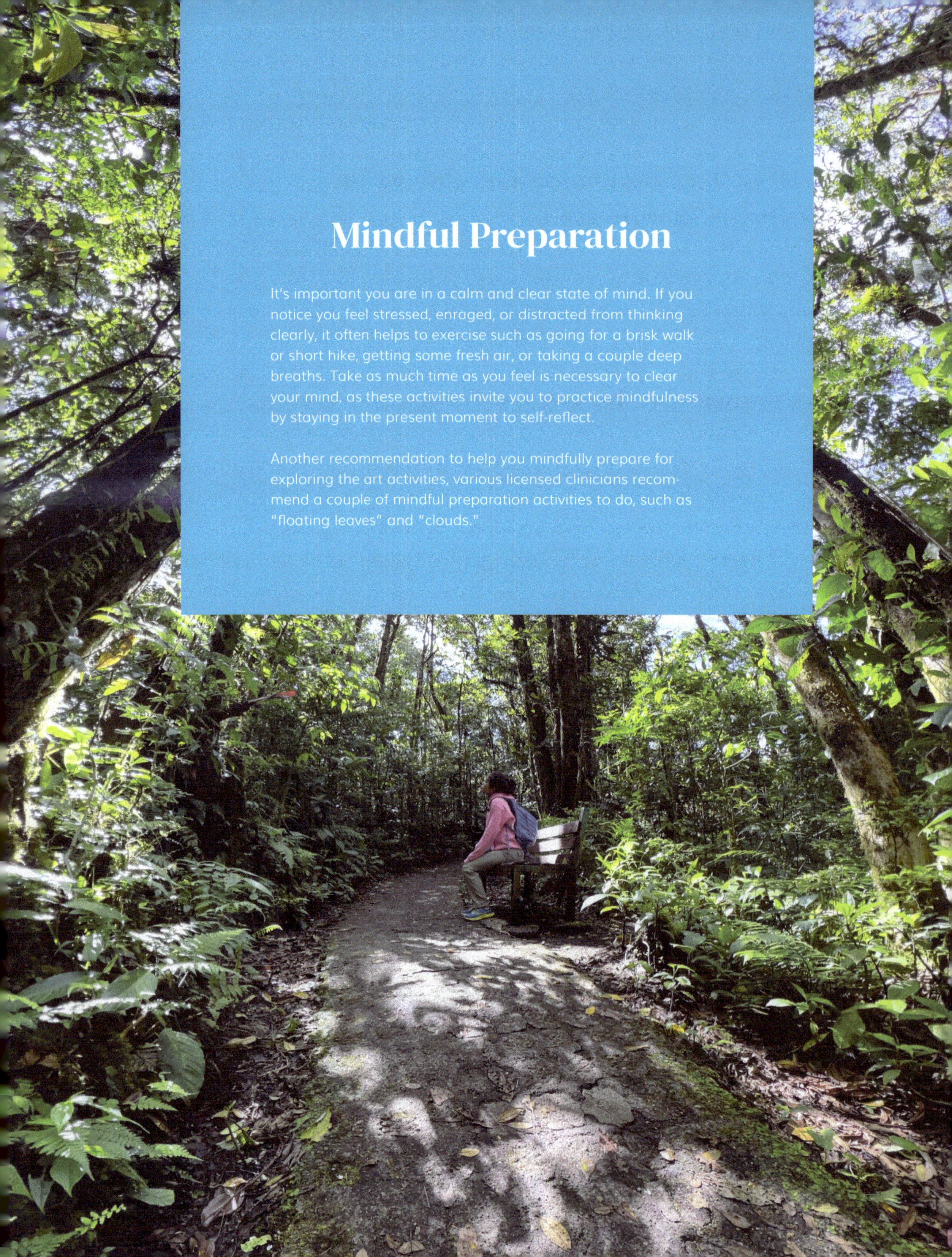

Mindful Preparation

It's important you are in a calm and clear state of mind. If you notice you feel stressed, enraged, or distracted from thinking clearly, it often helps to exercise such as going for a brisk walk or short hike, getting some fresh air, or taking a couple deep breaths. Take as much time as you feel is necessary to clear your mind, as these activities invite you to practice mindfulness by staying in the present moment to self-reflect.

Another recommendation to help you mindfully prepare for exploring the art activities, various licensed clinicians recommend a couple of mindful preparation activities to do, such as "floating leaves" and "clouds."

Preparation Exercise 1

Floating Leaves Guided Meditation Walkthrough:
A Meditation On Letting Go Of Control

Read through this meditation before practicing it, or find someone to read it to you, in a calm and gentle voice. If you're by yourself, set a timer for five minutes. If someone is reading it to you, make sure that they pause in between the prompts.

When you're ready...

> *Sit down with both of your feet on the ground, or lie down on your couch, bed, or a comfortable spot on the floor.*
>
> *Take a few deep breaths, in through your nose, pausing, and then out through your mouth.*
>
> *Not forcing anything, just letting your breath feel heavy and slow.*
>
> *And then let your breath return to normal.*
>
> *Our minds are always chattering away.*
>
> *Some people call our minds "monkey minds," because they're always reaching for the next thought. So for today's meditation, instead of focusing on stopping thoughts, or making thoughts disappear, we are just going to focus on letting thoughts go.*
>
> *Imagine you're standing in front of a creek, or a stream.*
>
> *Anytime a thought comes up for you, I want you to take that thought, put that thought on a leaf, put the leaf on the creek, and let the thought gently float away.*
>
> *Any kind of thought at all.*
>
> *Take that thought, place that thought on a leaf, place the leaf on the creek, and let the thought gently float away.*
>
> *[pause]*
>
> *You might notice thoughts about what's coming up next, or what else you have to do today...*

but as soon as you notice that thought, take the thought, place that thought on a leaf, place the leaf on the creek, and let the thought gently float away.

[pause]

You may have thoughts come up and bring up other emotions, like stress, or anger, or anxiety.

And of course, thoughts aren't in charge of our feelings, we are, so as soon as you notice that thought, take the thought, place that thought on a leaf, place the leaf on the creek, and let the thought gently float away.

[pause]

Some thoughts feel kind of sticky.

They come up again, and again, and again.

But as soon as you notice that thought, take the thought, place that thought on a leaf, place the leaf on the creek, and let the thought gently float away. And if you notice the thought comes up again, take the thought, place that thought on a leaf, place the leaf on the creek, and let the thought gently float away.

[pause]

You might notice thoughts about different sounds or sensations around you.

As soon as you notice the thought, take the thought, place that thought on a leaf, place the leaf on the creek, and let the thought gently float away.

[pause]

You might notice a thought like, "How long do I have to do this meditation for?"

And as soon as you notice the thought, take the thought, place that thought on a leaf, place the leaf on the creek, and let the thought gently float away.

[pause]

Sometimes your mind will feel really quiet, and other times it will feel really loud with a thought.

So as soon as you notice the thought, take the thought, place that thought on a leaf, place the leaf on the creek, and let the thought gently float away.

[pause]
We'll stay here for a few more moments.

Noticing thoughts, placing the thoughts on leaves, placing the leaves on the creek, and letting the leaves gently float away.

[Remain in this quiet space, aiming for 5 minutes of meditation the first time, and then building to 10-15 minutes on subsequent meditation practices]

Remember, meditation for anxiety is a practice, not a destination.

We don't just automatically become great at meditation. We need to do it regularly to become good at it.

We also want to practice acceptance of our difficulties with meditation. It's ok if your thoughts feel really loud and hard to move away from! The more you practice, the easier it will be - but it's always ok if you hit a bump in the road, too.

The best way to improve your meditation is to set up a regular time each week to practice. Some people love to meditate before bed, others take a five-minute meditation break before homework, and some people say that Saturday is their meditation day, and they'll practice every Saturday afternoon.

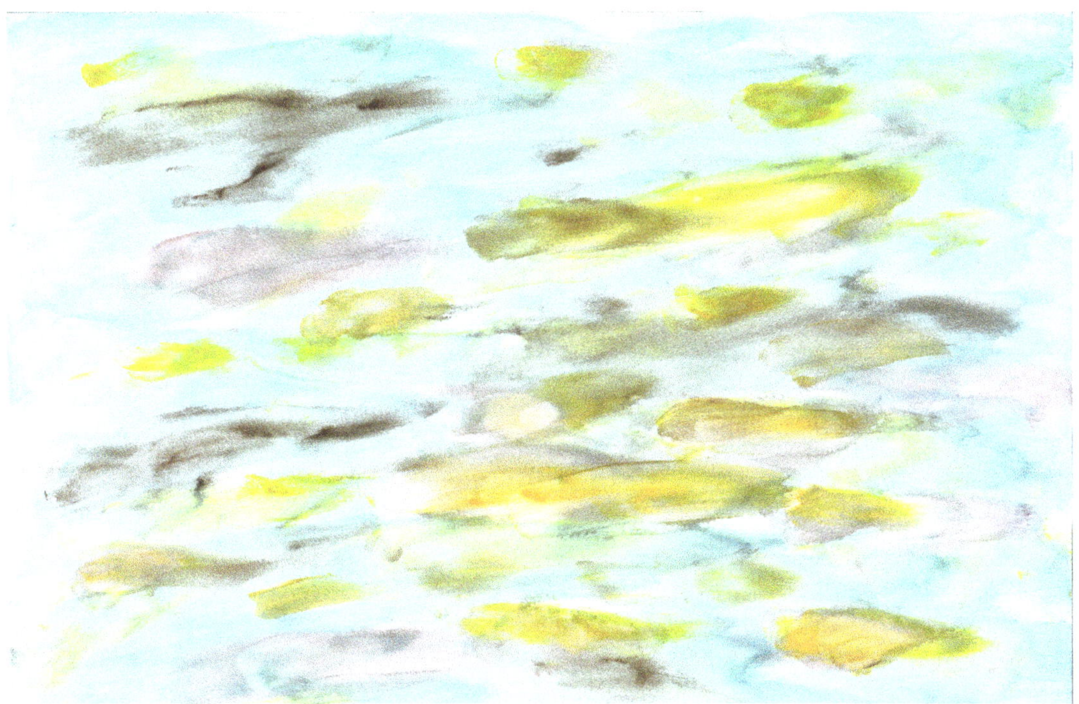

Preparation Exercise 2

Clouds Mindfulness Practice

Sit up tall, close your eyes, and place your hands on your knees. Begin to take a nice, long, slow, deep breath in ~ As you inhale, imagine you are breathing in a big comforting cloud of love and happiness inside your heart, and every time you breathe in more and more again, it gets bigger and more calming! Now, remain still and breathe out a nice, long, slow breath, letting go of any worries.

Enjoy the warm feeling of comfort, love, and joy surrounding you and within you.

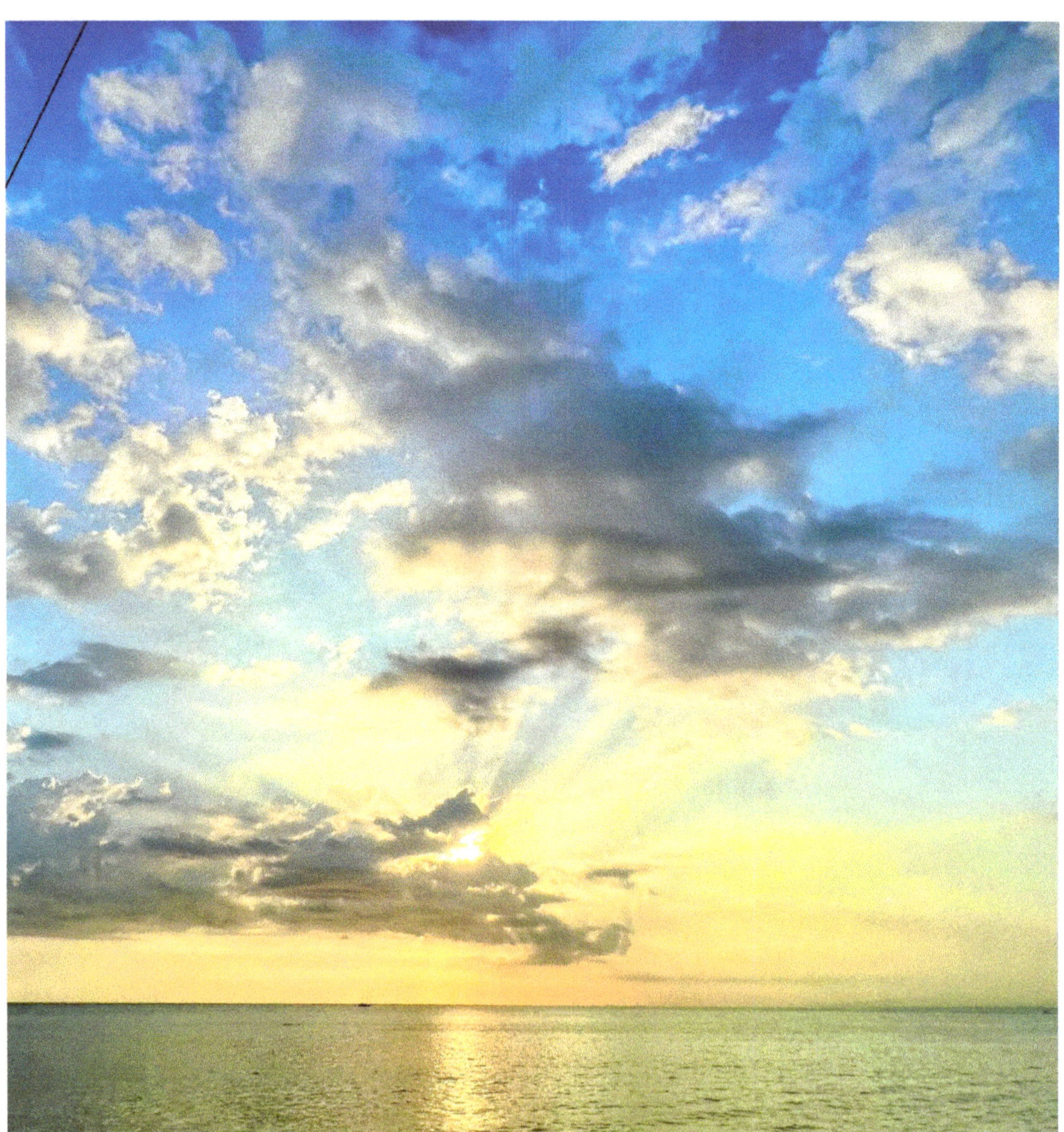

Chapter 1:
All About You

"The aim of art is to represent not the outward appearance of things, but their inward significance."

– Aristotle

The Mind-Body Connection

Art therapy is using art to express yourself, explore your feelings, and heal. It recognizes that our mental well-being is connected to our bodies and emotions. Creating art helps you show what's inside, understand your emotions, and become more self-aware.

These exercises presented to you in this chapter serve as a means of self-reflection, as anxiety can often be very physical (i.e., sweaty palms, rapid heart rate, difficulty sleeping, etc.). When you are able to pay attention to what places, people, or events make you feel anxious, it's easier to find healthy coping techniques to manage your anxiety before or during those events. Having a sense of control warps the anxiety trigger and makes it smaller and more manageable.

Art therapy lets you get in touch with the physical manifestations of anxiety and express things you might find hard to say with words. Making art taps into your creativity and lets you safely express yourself. I hope you find the following exercises valuable in your journey toward emotional well-being.

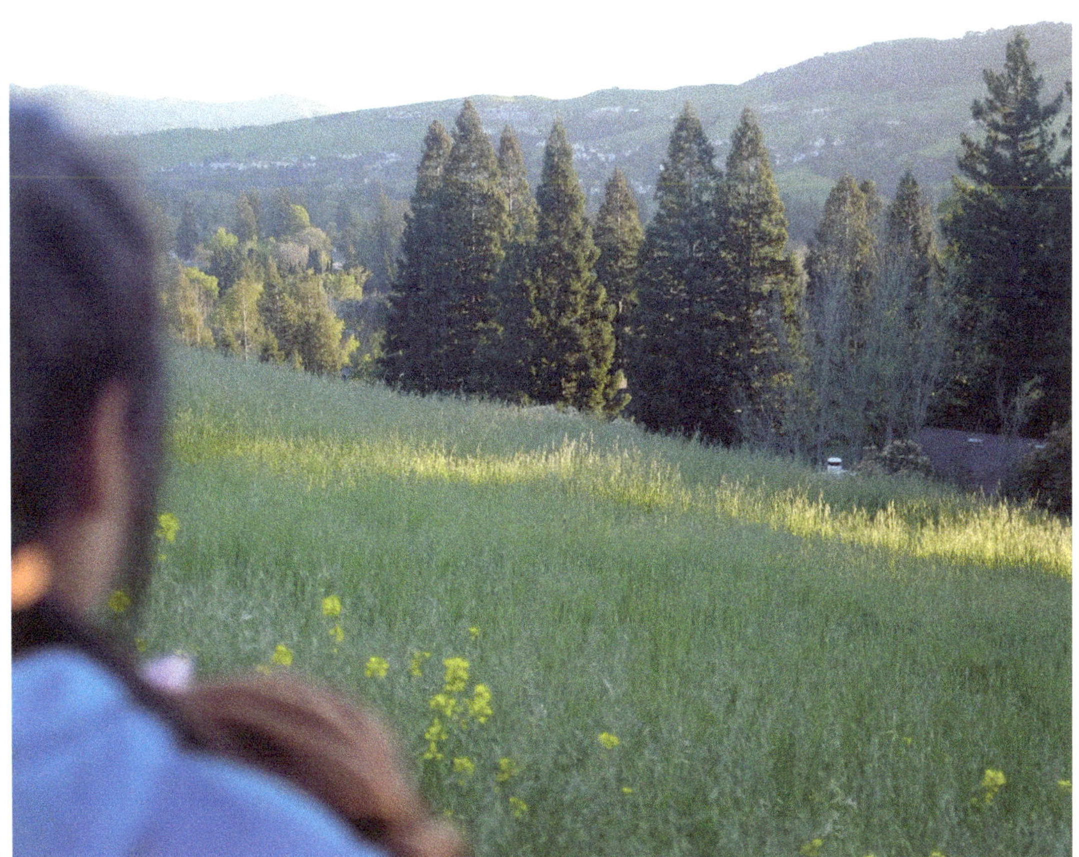

Breath-Flow Doodles

Grab a piece of paper and some colored markers. Start by taking a few deep breaths to calm your mind. As you breathe in and out, let your hand move across the paper, creating doodles and patterns that match the rhythm of your breath. It's like turning your breath into art!

Sensory Self-Portrait Journey

Imagine you're an artist-adventurer exploring your own body. As you create a self-portrait, think about how each part of your body feels. Use different textures and colors to capture those sensations. It's like making a map of your inner landscape.

Nature Sensation Art

Head to a nearby park or green space. Close your eyes, breathe in the fresh air, and feel the ground beneath your feet. Collect leaves, rocks, or sticks, and use them to create an artwork that reflects your nature adventure. It's like bringing a piece of the outdoors into your art.

Chakra Art Exploration

Chakras energy centers inside us that are linked to our physical, mental, and spiritual well-being. These chakras are rooted in ancient Indian traditions like Hinduism and Buddhism. The word 'chakra' actually means 'wheel' or 'disk' in Sanskrit, and it's like they're these spinning wheels of energy.

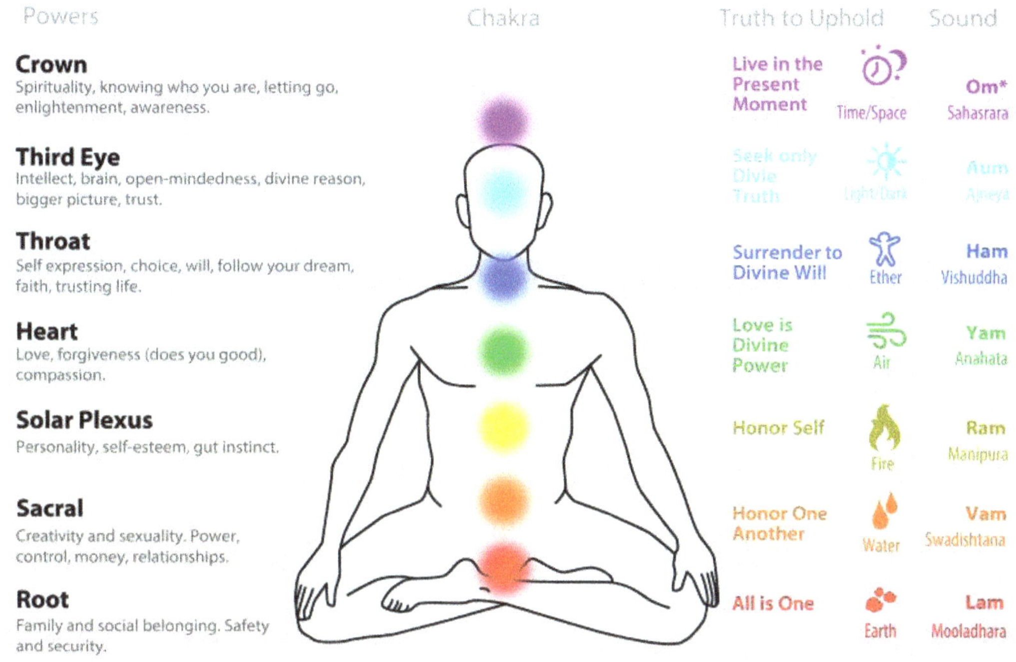

Credit: Amber Urman

Each chakra illustrated[5] above is believed to be connected to specific parts of our lives, like our feelings, thoughts, and our health. When these chakras are in harmony, there is a smooth energy flow and that has a positive effect on us. But when there are imbalances in these chakras, it can negatively affect our physical and emotional health.

---

[5] smallripples.com

I KNOW

I SEE

I SPEAK

I LOVE

I DO

I FEEL

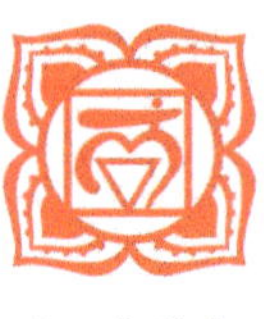

I AM

CROWN CHAKRA

DIVINE CONNECTION | CONSCIOUSNESS | ENGLIGHTENMENT

I am connected to the Divine and acknowledge my own Divinity.

THIRD EYE CHAKRA

INTUITION | WISDOM | IMAGINATION | DREAMS

I listen to the guidance of my intuition and follow its wisdom.

THROAT CHAKRA

SELF-EXPRESSION | COMMUNICATION | AUTHENTICITY

I am confident in expressing myself and in communicating my ideas.

HEART CHAKRA

UNCONDITIONAL LOVE | COMPASSION | EMPATHY

I practice unconditional love towards myself and towards others.

SOLAR PLEXUS CHAKRA

ACTION | PERSONAL POWER | CONFIDENCE

I am powerful and confident and determined to make my dreams a reality.

SACRAL CHAKRA

CREATIVITY | SEXUALITY | PLEASURE | EMOTIONS

I feel my emotions deeply and explore my creativity and sexuality.

ROOT CHAKRA

IDENTITY | STABILITY | SECURITY | EARTHLY

I am grounded and my roots are firmly connected to the earth.

[5] smallripples.com

In art therapy, we can use the chakra system as a roadmap to understand and manage our anxiety. Here is one way to do it:

1. **Identify the Affected Chakra(s)**: You'll want to think about which chakras are linked to the feelings and issues connected to your anxiety. Maybe it's the Root Chakra (all about feeling safe) or the Solar Plexus Chakra (all about self-esteem and confidence).

2. **Mindful Exploration**: Start with some mindfulness exercises or guided meditation to get you in tune with your anxiety and where you feel it in your body.

3. **Art Materials**: Grab your art supplies—colored pencils, paints, whatever you like. You can also pick colors that match the chakras. It's a cool way to kick things off.

4. **Chakra-Inspired Art**: Make some art that shows how you're feeling right now. Use colors, shapes, and symbols that fit your mood, based on the chakra connected to your anxiety. It's like a visual diary of your emotions. You can also use the chakra templates provided in the Art Therapy Templates section of this book.

5. **Let It Out Through Art**: Creating art is like giving your feelings a voice without words. It can help you let go of built-up emotions and give you insights into what's going on inside.

6. **Reflect and Understand**: After your artwork is done, think about what you've made. Journal about how your colors, shapes, and symbols connect to your anxiety and feeling.

7. **Find Balance and Healing**: Work on balancing the affected chakra(s). You can set goals for self-improvement or try out other art therapy methods to feel better and more relaxed.

8. **Continued Exploration**: Art therapy isn't a one-time exercise. I encourage you to keep going with it, track your progress, and dive deeper into your anxiety.

Using chakras in art therapy to tackle anxiety is like turning your feelings into art and finding your inner balance along the way.

Crown Chakra ("I Know")

I am connected to the Divine and acknowledge my own Divinity.

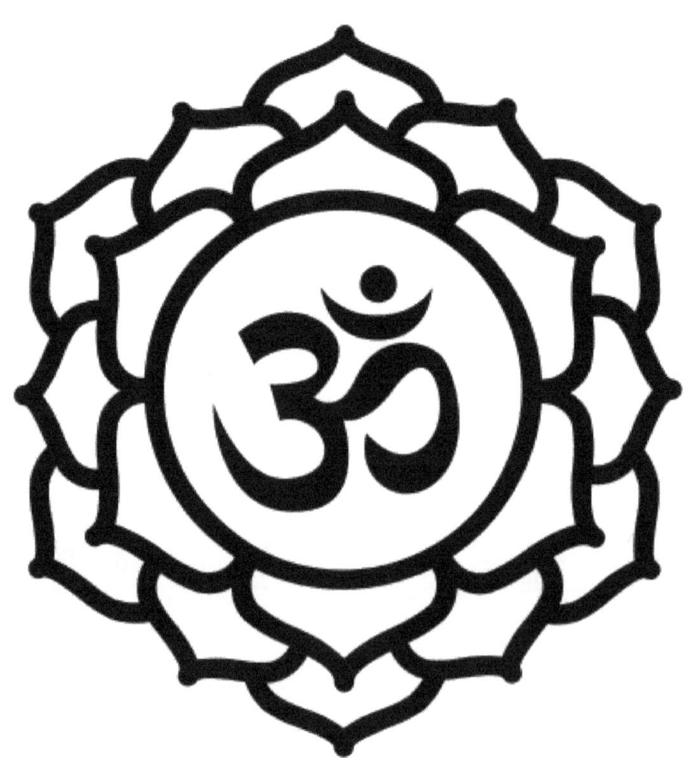

Third Eye Chakra("I See")

I listen to the guidance of my intuition and follow its wisdom.

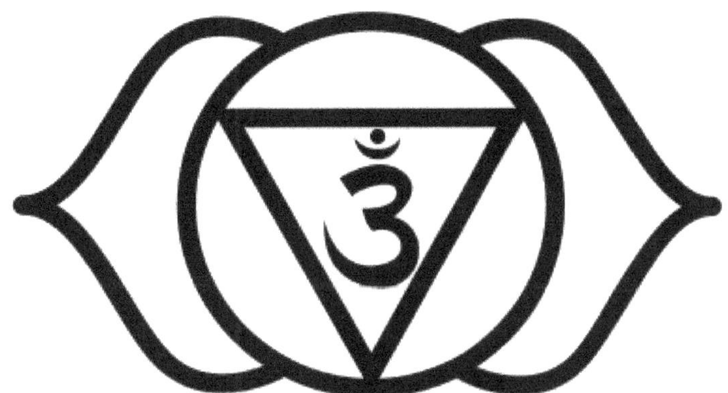

Throat Chakra ("I Speak")

I am confident in expressing myself and in communicating my ideas.

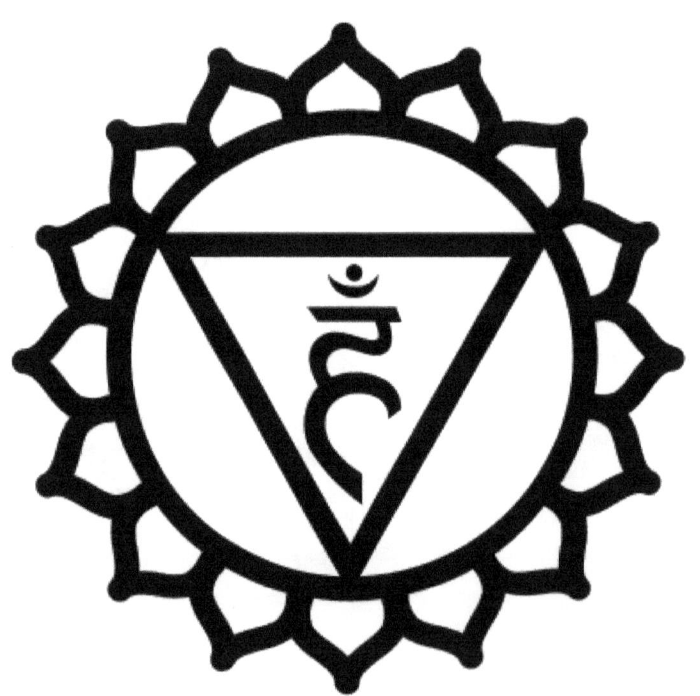

Heart Chakra ("I Love")

I practice unconditional love towards myself and towards others.

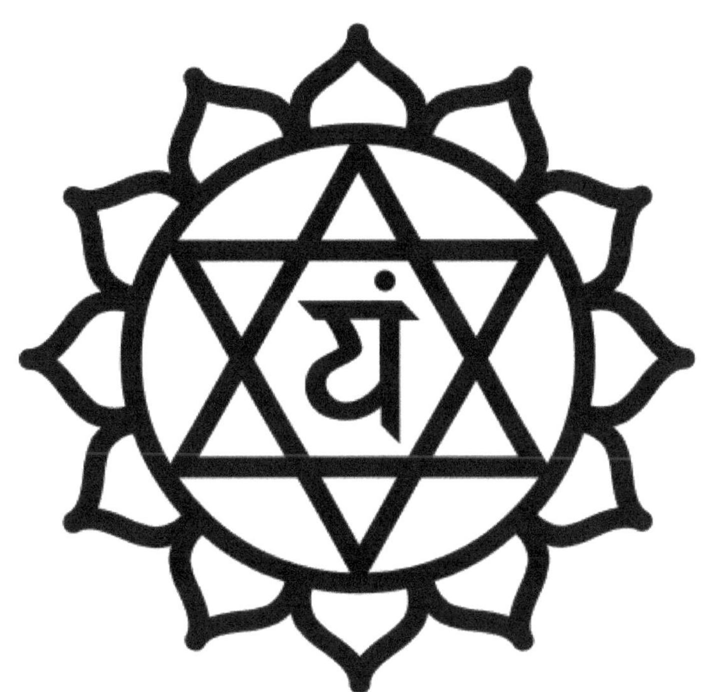

Solar Plexus Chakra ("I Do")

I am powerful and confident and determined to
make my dreams a reality.

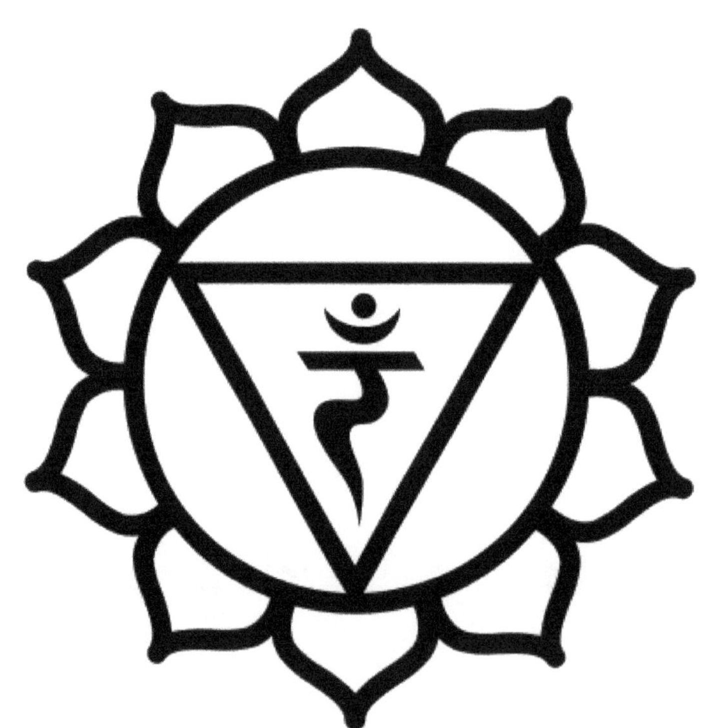

Sacral Chakra ("I Feel")

I feel my emotions deeply and explore my creativity and sexuality.

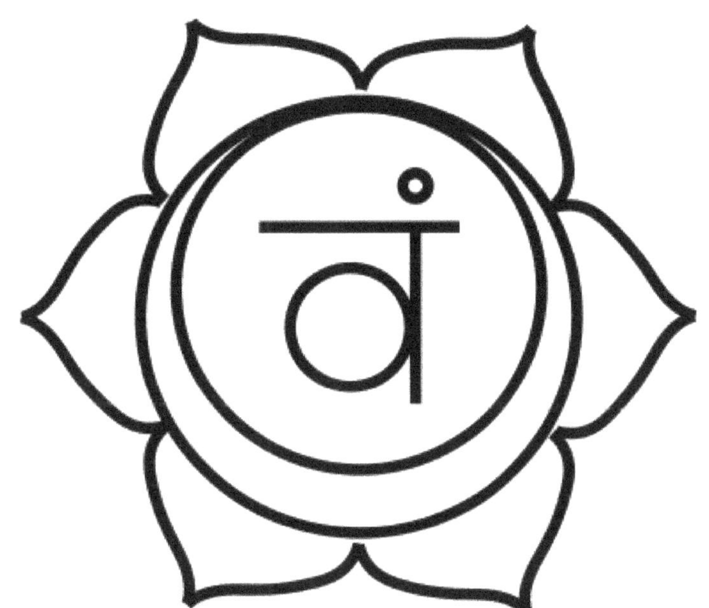

Root Chakra ("I Am")

I am grounded and my roots are firmly connected to the earth.

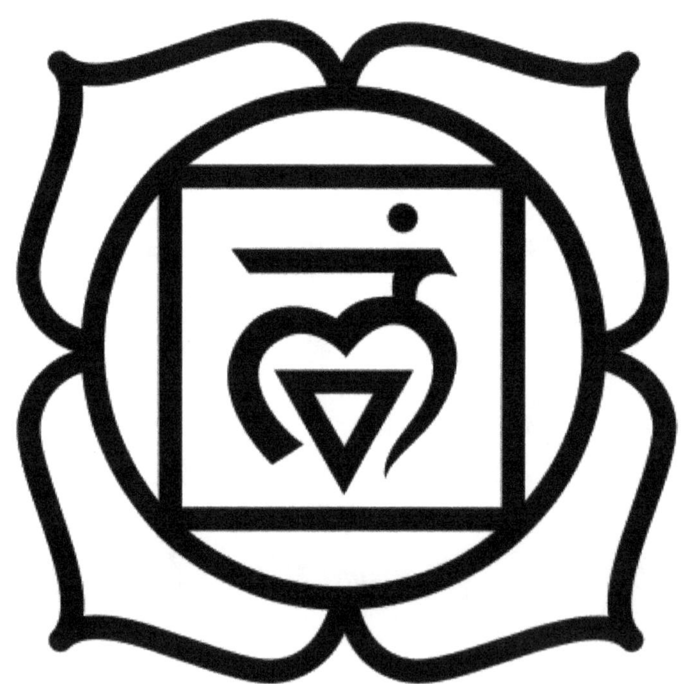

Emotion Wheel

An 'emotion wheel' is a helpful tool in art therapy that helps us deal with our feelings. The goal of the emotion wheel exercises is to help you identify feelings - for me, naming an emotion helps me feel in control.

Now, imagine it as a colorful circle with sections. Each section represents a different color and each individual color represents a different emotion. It's a creative way to express and understand our emotions, relax, and think about what's going on inside. Plus, we can share our artwork with others to help them understand our feelings better. So, the 'emotion wheel' is like our personal guide to understanding and expressing our feelings in a fun and creative way.

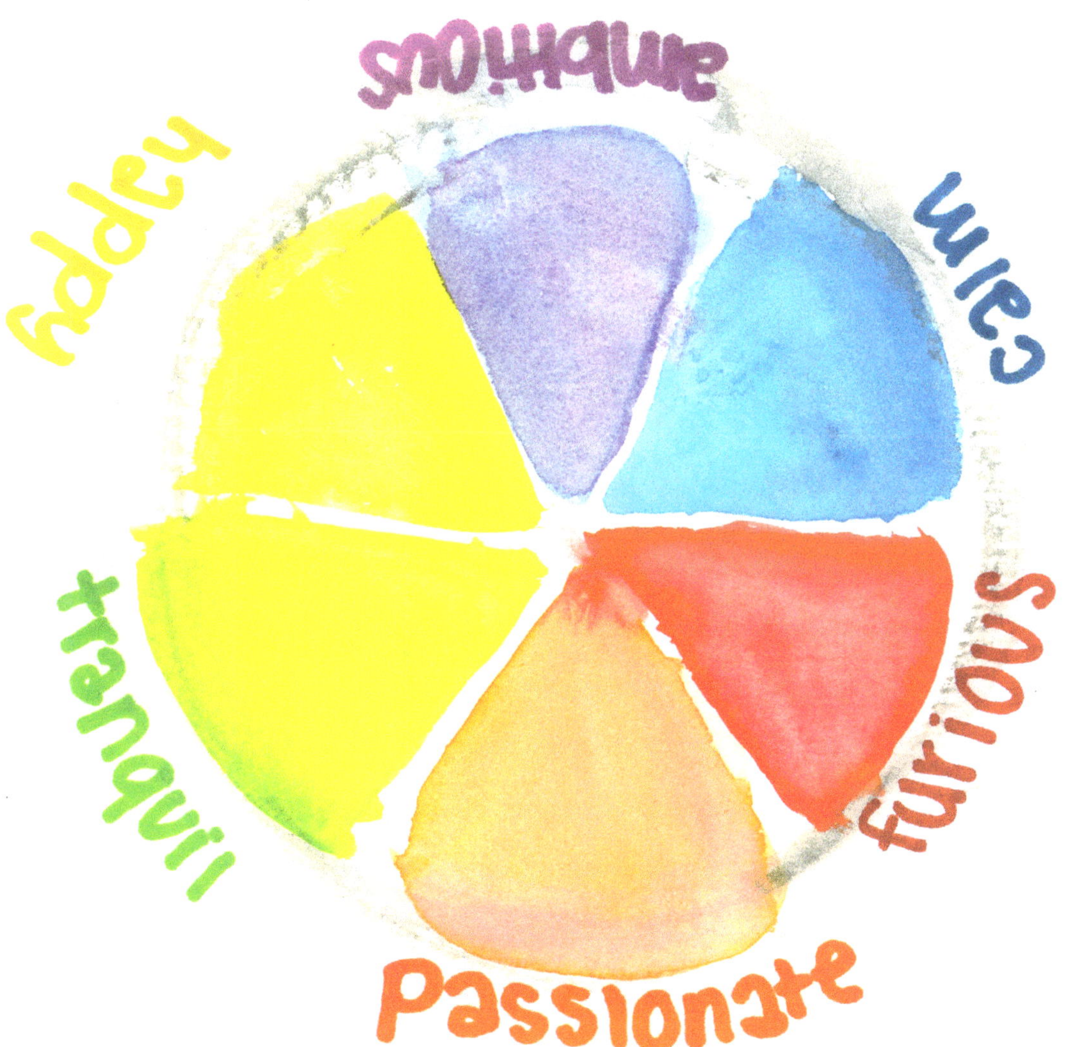

Emoji Emotion Wheel

Grab a big piece of paper and draw a giant circle in the center. Divide the circle into slices, like a pizza, and label each slice with an emotion: happy, sad, angry, surprised, scared, and calm. Now, it's emoji time! Draw or paste emojis that match each emotion in its slice. Color and decorate it with your own style. You've just created your very own emoji emotion wheel! It's like making your personal emoji mood chart.

Feeling Collage

Get some old magazines or print out pictures from the internet. Cut out images or words that represent different emotions like joy, frustration, excitement, or peace. Arrange and glue them onto a big piece of paper to create a colorful collage. When you're done, talk with your friends about what emotions you included and why. It's like making a collage of your feelings!

Color Your Emotions

Take a blank emotion wheel template or draw one yourself with different emotions around the circle. Now, it's time to color! Use crayons, colored pencils, or markers to fill in each emotion section with a color that matches how you feel when experiencing that emotion. Share your colorful emotion wheel with your friends and ask them what colors they would choose.

Storyboard of Emotions

Imagine you're creating a comic book or storyboard. Draw a series of pictures that show a little story about how you might feel in different situations. For example, a scene of you being excited to see your friends, or a moment when you're feeling a bit down. Write short captions or dialog bubbles to explain each emotion. Share your storyboard with friends, and maybe even turn it into a group storytelling activity. It's like making your own mini emotions comic book!

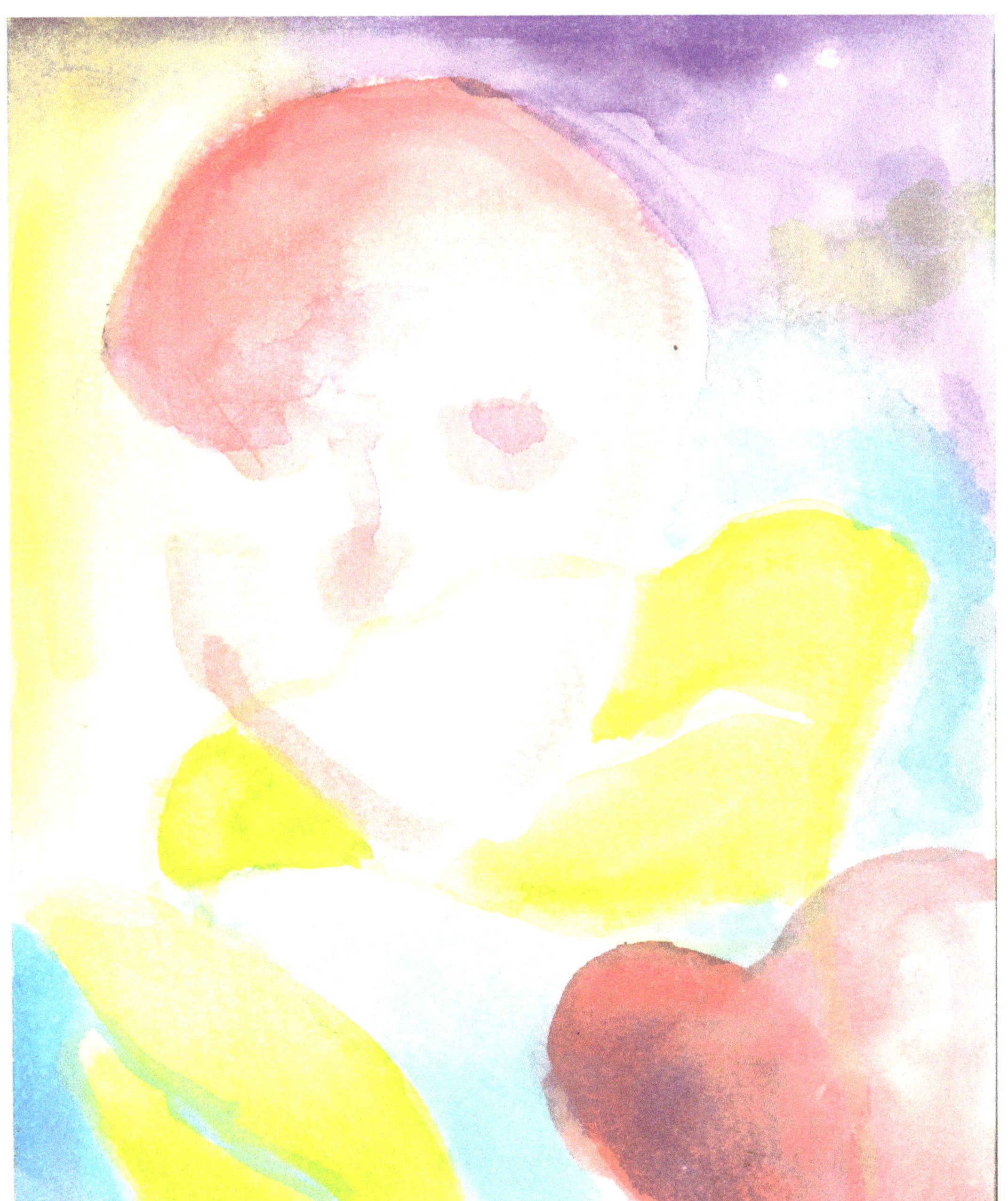

Storyboard Template

Feelings Wheel Paintings

Use watercolors or acrylic paints to create a circular painting. Divide the circle into sections and write an emotion in each section. Paint each section with colors that express how that emotion feels to you. Use brushes, sponges, or your fingers to create different textures. Hang up your feelings wheel painting in your room as a reminder of your emotions and how they can be beautiful and colorful!

Mountain and Valley Metaphor

The 'mountain and valley metaphor' is like a visual way of understanding our emotions in art therapy. When we're feeling great, we draw a colorful mountain to represent when we're feeling our best. But when we're facing tough times, we sketch a valley to represent those challenges. We can get creative with our drawings, adding details like sunshine or clouds. This helps us reflect on our feelings and understand our emotional ups and downs. It's like creating a personal emotional map and realizing that life is a mix of highs and lows, aiming for balance in our emotional landscape.

Visualizing your vast array of emotions you experience daily allows you to gain a more enhanced sense of self awareness and understanding that both the positive and negative feelings you experience are normal and make you human.

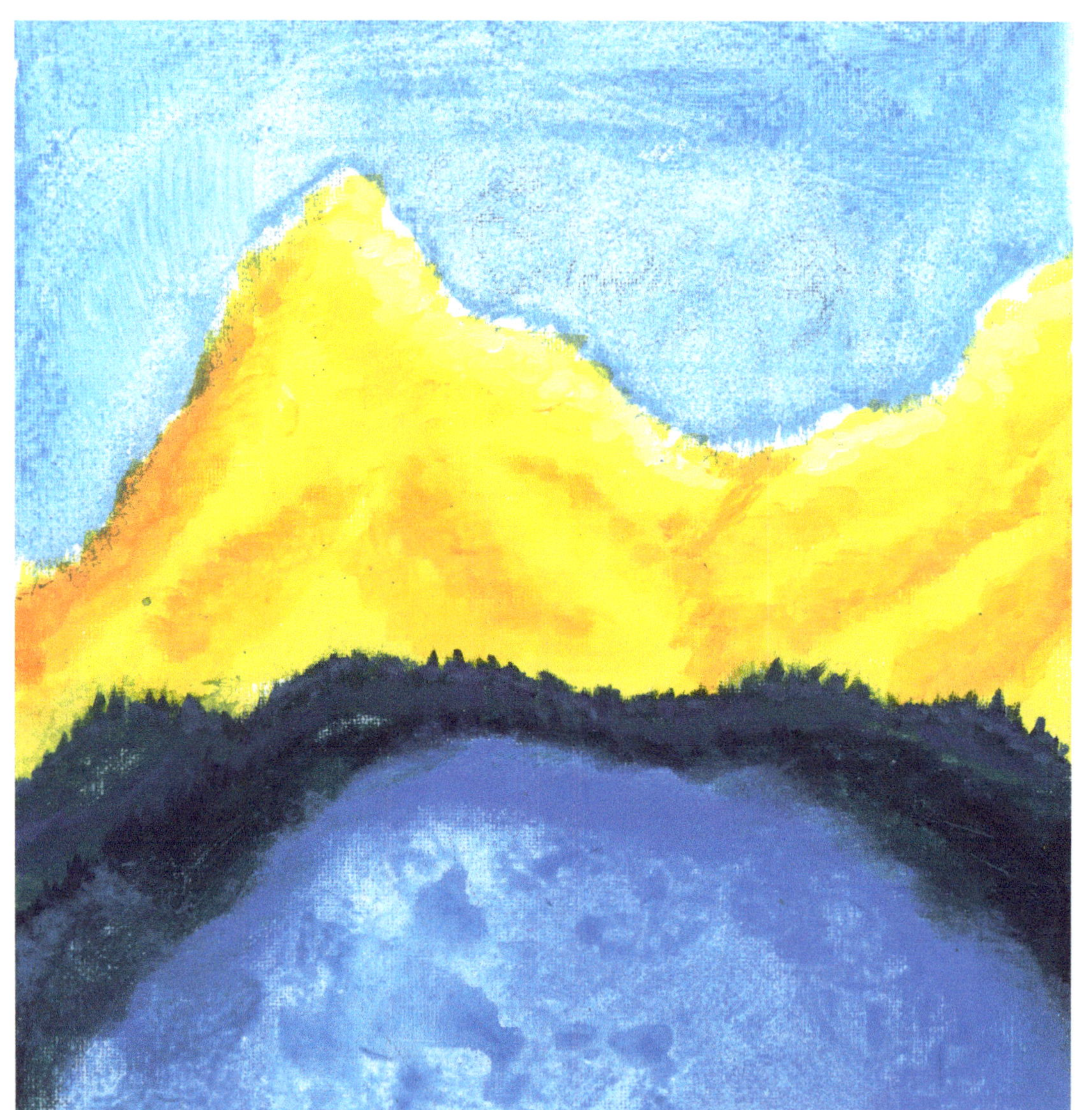

Peaks and Pits Painting

Start with a blank canvas or paper. Think of the "peaks" as the best moments or highlights in your life so far, and the "pits" as the challenging or low points.

- Paint a mountain with peaks and valleys to represent these moments. Use bright colors for the peaks and darker shades for the valleys.
- You can even write short descriptions or draw symbols to represent specific events or feelings associated with each peak and pit.
- Share your artwork with friends and discuss your own mountains and valleys. It's like creating a visual timeline of your life's ups and downs!

Emotion Elevation Collage

Collect magazines, newspapers, or print out images from the internet. Find pictures that represent different emotions you've experienced recently.

- Create a collage on a poster board or paper. Arrange the emotions like a mountain range, with the most intense emotions at the peaks and the milder ones in the valleys.
- Add captions or words to describe how you felt during each emotion.
- Share your emotion elevation collage with your friends and ask them to create their own. It's like making a collage of your emotional journey!

Personal Growth Landscape

Imagine the mountain as your personal growth journey, and the valley as any obstacles or challenges you've faced.

- Draw or paint a landscape with a mountain in the background and a valley in the foreground.
- Decorate the mountain with symbols or images representing your achievements, goals, or dreams. Decorate the valley with things that symbolize challenges you've overcome or are currently facing.
- Reflect on how you've grown and learned from your experiences and share your artwork and insights with friends.

Chapter 2:
Calming & Relaxation

*"Art is my cure to all this madness, sadness and loss of belonging
in the world and through it I'll walk myself home."*

– Nikki Rowe

"Calming and visualization" art therapy exercises are creative ways to find your tranquility. Through art, you can relax, reduce stress, and feel peaceful. Imagine painting soothing colors, creating intricate designs with Zentangles, or picturing a tranquil scene in your mind while you draw. These exercises help you combine the power of art and visualization to create a sense of calm and relaxation, making it easier to cope with life's ups and downs. It's like painting your worries away and finding a peaceful oasis in your creative world. When you are calm and relaxed, it's easier to stay in the present moment without multitasking your overwhelming emotions.

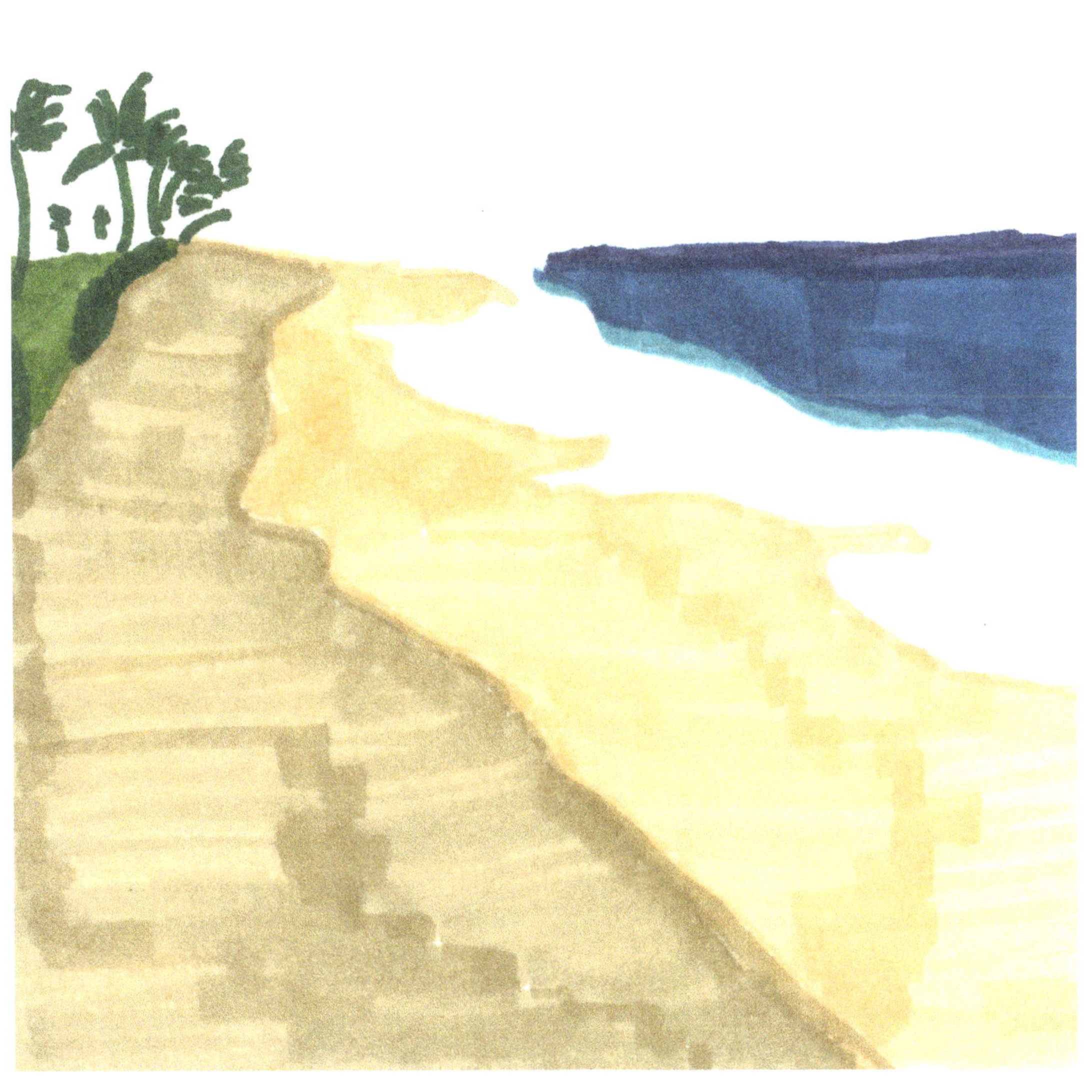

Zen-tangle Your Stress Away

Creating a zentangle involves drawing a "tangle" of lines that are then filled with repetitive patterns or designs. Each zentangle is unique...as you are the one making the tangle of lines and choosing the patterns to fill the voids with.

- Get a piece of paper and a fine-tip pen.
- Start with a small, simple shape or design in the center of your paper.
- Fill the rest of the paper with intricate, repetitive patterns, like swirls, dots, and lines. Let your pen flow with calm, steady movements.
- Focus on your breathing as you create your zen-tangle art. It's like a mindful meditation in art form. Share your zen-tangle creation with your friends and encourage them to try it too. It's like doodling your worries away!

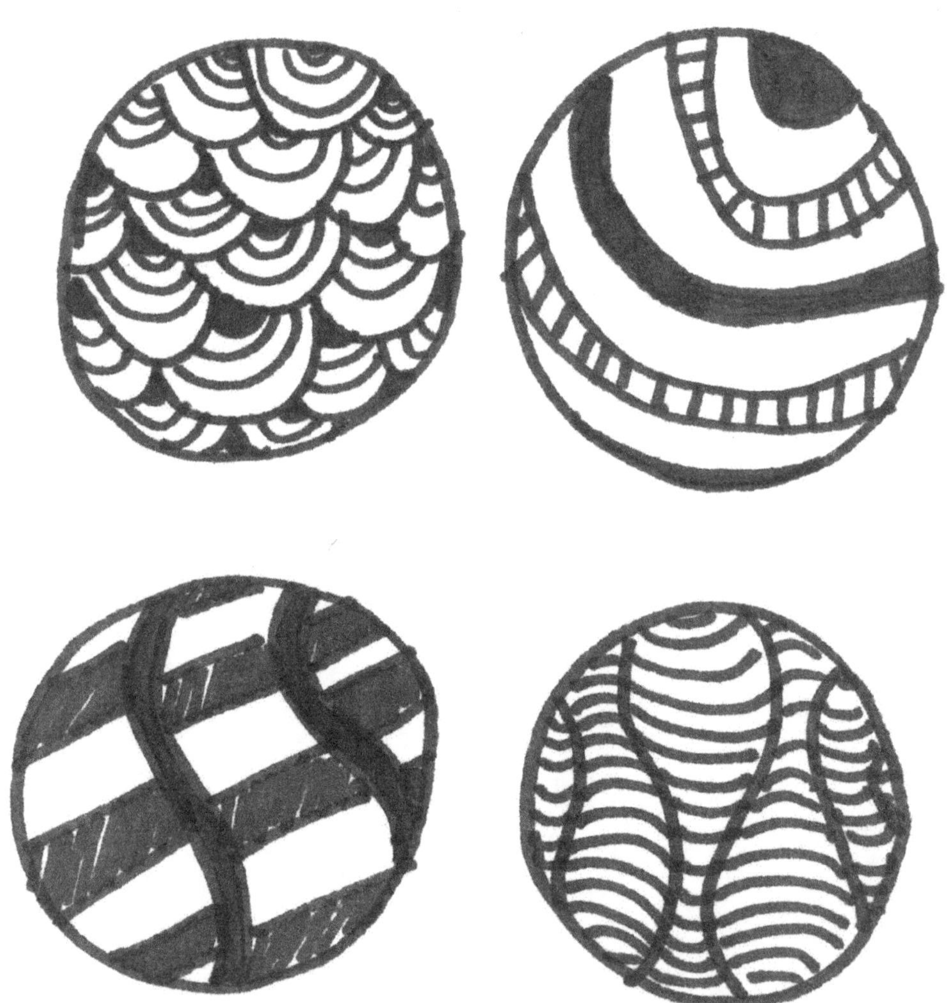

Finger Paint Freedom

Find some finger paints or acrylic paints. Forget about brushes!

- Dip your fingers right into the paint and let your hands roam freely on the canvas or paper. Close your eyes if it helps you relax. Explore the tactile sensation of the paint on your fingers and the canvas.
- Create abstract patterns or even a soothing landscape with just your fingertips.
- Share your finger-painted masterpiece with your friends and chat about how it felt to get your hands messy in a calming way.

Colorful Calm Palette

Choose a color palette that soothes you. It could be soft pastels, gentle blues and greens, or any combination that makes you feel relaxed.

- Create an artwork using only those calming colors. Paint a serene scene, an abstract pattern, or anything that comes to mind.
- Let the colors wash over you like a wave of calmness.
- Share your calming color artwork with your friends and ask them which colors make them feel most relaxed. It's like painting with your peaceful palette!

Guided Relaxation Art

Find a guided relaxation audio online or use a meditation app.

- Listen to the soothing voice as it leads you through a relaxation exercise.
- While you listen, create art that reflects the imagery and feelings from the guided relaxation. You can use watercolors, colored pencils, or any art supplies you like.
- Share your relaxation art with your friends and discuss how the guided meditation helped you create a sense of calm through your artwork. It's like painting your peaceful journey!

Art and Music

Draw, scribble, or paint to your favorite song. Feel free to illustrate your emotions on paper or a canvas or recreate an image that resonates with you.

Chapter 3: Visualization

"The moods and qualities of nature and the revelations of great art are difficult to define; we can grasp them only in the depths of our perceptive spirit."

– Ansel Adams

Visualization exercises in art therapy involve using your imagination to create mental images that help you explore and express your emotions and thoughts. But more importantly, visualization helps you to create a safe space for your mind before or when you begin to experience feelings of anxiety. Being able to visualize a safe space helps you to reset your mind and regulate your emotions. So when you return back to the place you are in, you can be present in the activity you're doing or the people you are socializing with without being distracted by your negative emotions.

You can also think about it as daydreaming with a purpose. You can close your eyes and picture something that represents your feelings or experiences, then use art to bring that mental image to life. This exercise turns your thoughts and emotions into a personal artwork, making it easier to understand and process your feelings in a visual and meaningful way.

Dreamscape Painting

Close your eyes and visualize a peaceful or happy place then paint or draw that mental image.

Emotion Collage

Collect images from magazines or printouts that represent various emotions. Create a collage that reflects your emotional journey. This activity can be a powerful way to explore and understand your feelings.

Guided Imagery Painting

Listen to a guided meditation or visualization audio and paint or draw what you imagine during the session.

Self-Portrait Evolution

Create a series of self-portraits that show your emotional evolution over time. Start with a self-portrait that represents your current emotional state and then create additional portraits and regular intervals (e.g. monthly) to track changes.

Inner Landscape

Close your eyes and visualize your inner world or inner landscape. What does it look like? What elements are present? Create a piece of art based on this visualization to gain insight into your inner self.

"I am" Collage

Assemble images of items, places, colors, animals, or feelings that capture how you see yourself.

Chapter 4:
Letting Go

*"If you're brave enough to say goodbye,
life will reward you with a new hello."*

– Paulo Coehlo

As you have explored all of your unique and wonderful emotions to learn how to make those overwhelming feelings feel smaller and more manageable, I now welcome you to explore letting some of those "sticky" negative feelings go. The purpose of these activities is to practice acknowledging how something or someone may have made you feel defeated or gloomy, but it's equally as important to know how to let those feelings go so they don't end up holding you down.

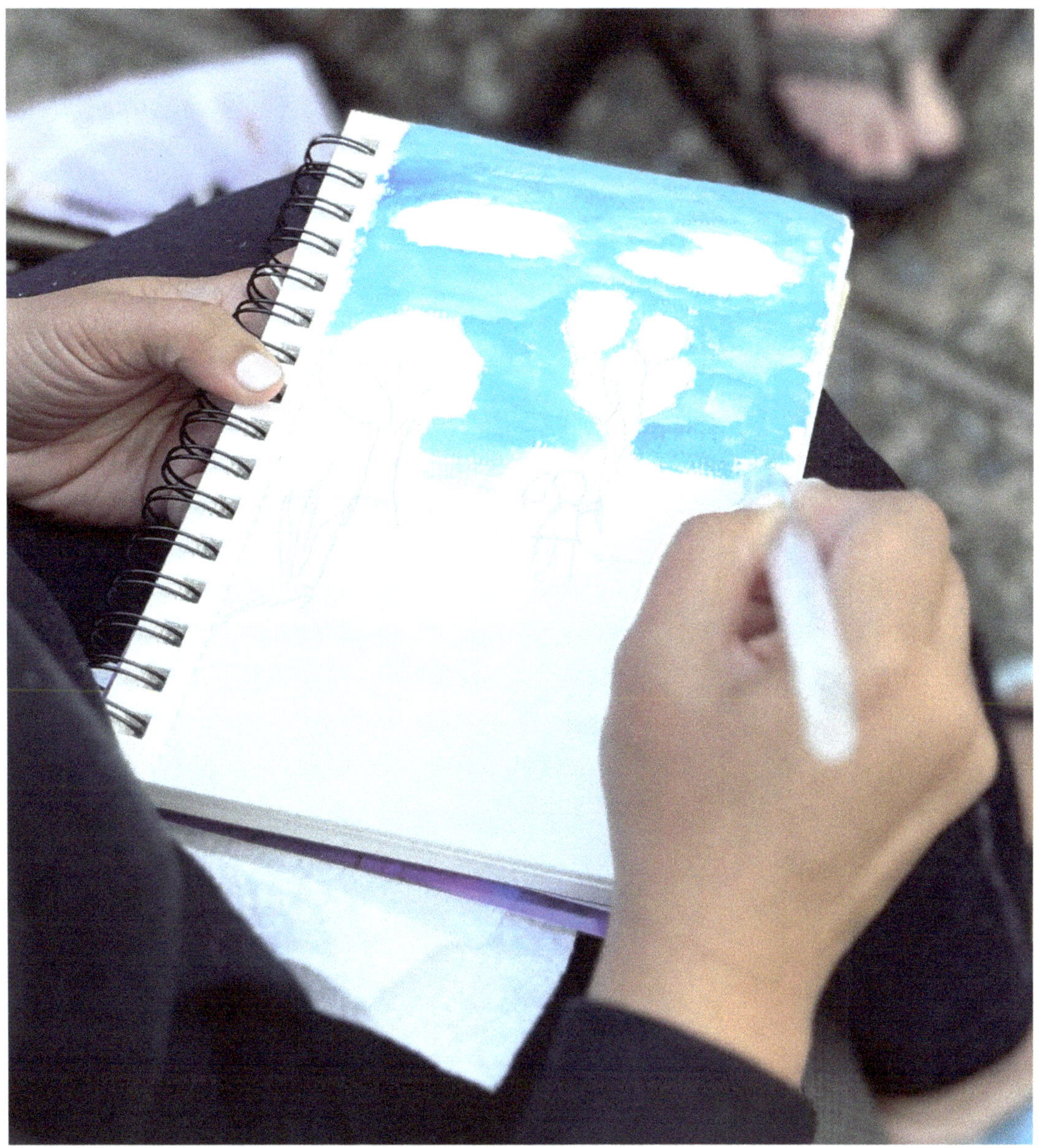

An important trait in letting go is forgiveness. When you can forgive someone, even if it's yourself, you are giving yourself permission to move forward and stop mourning over the past.

Balloon Message

In art therapy, the "balloon message" is a creative way to let go of worries and stress. Imagine drawing or writing down your worries on a piece of paper, then attaching it to a balloon. This activity helps you visualize your worries floating away which can bring a sense of relief and freedom. It's like a symbolic way to clear your mind and lighten your emotional load, leaving you with a sense of release and hope.

Balloon Message Art Journal

Start an art journal or a notebook.

- Whenever you have a strong emotion or thought, draw it or write it inside a "balloon" shape.
- Decorate the balloons with colors, patterns, or doodles that represent the feeling.
- Over time, your journal will be filled with these emotion balloons. Share your journal with your friends and encourage them to start their own.

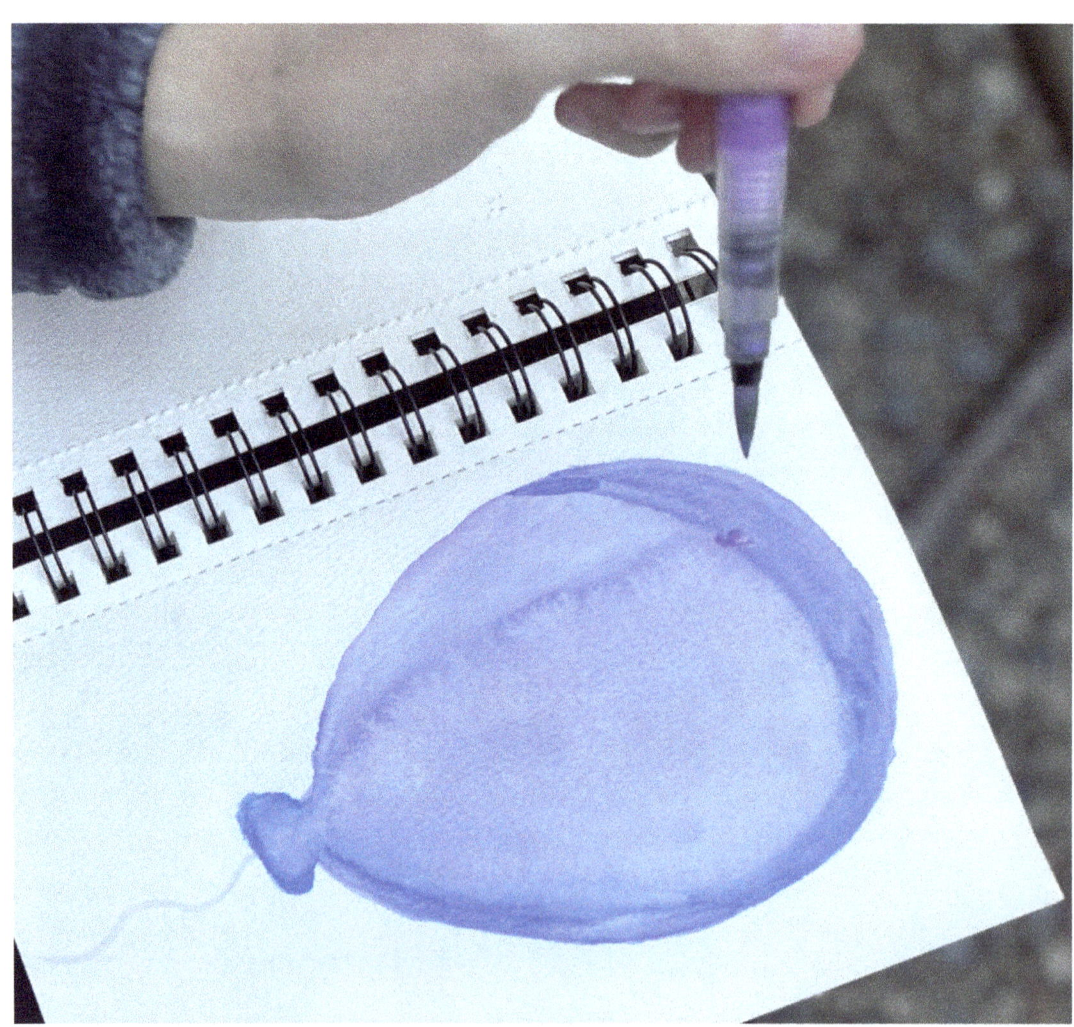

Balloon of Dreams

Draw or paint a big, colorful balloon on a sheet of paper.

- Inside the balloon, write or draw your dreams, goals, or your hopes in the future.
- Use bright and bold colors to make your dreams pop!
- Share your "balloon of dreams" with your friends and talk about your aspirations. It's like creating a visual bucket list!

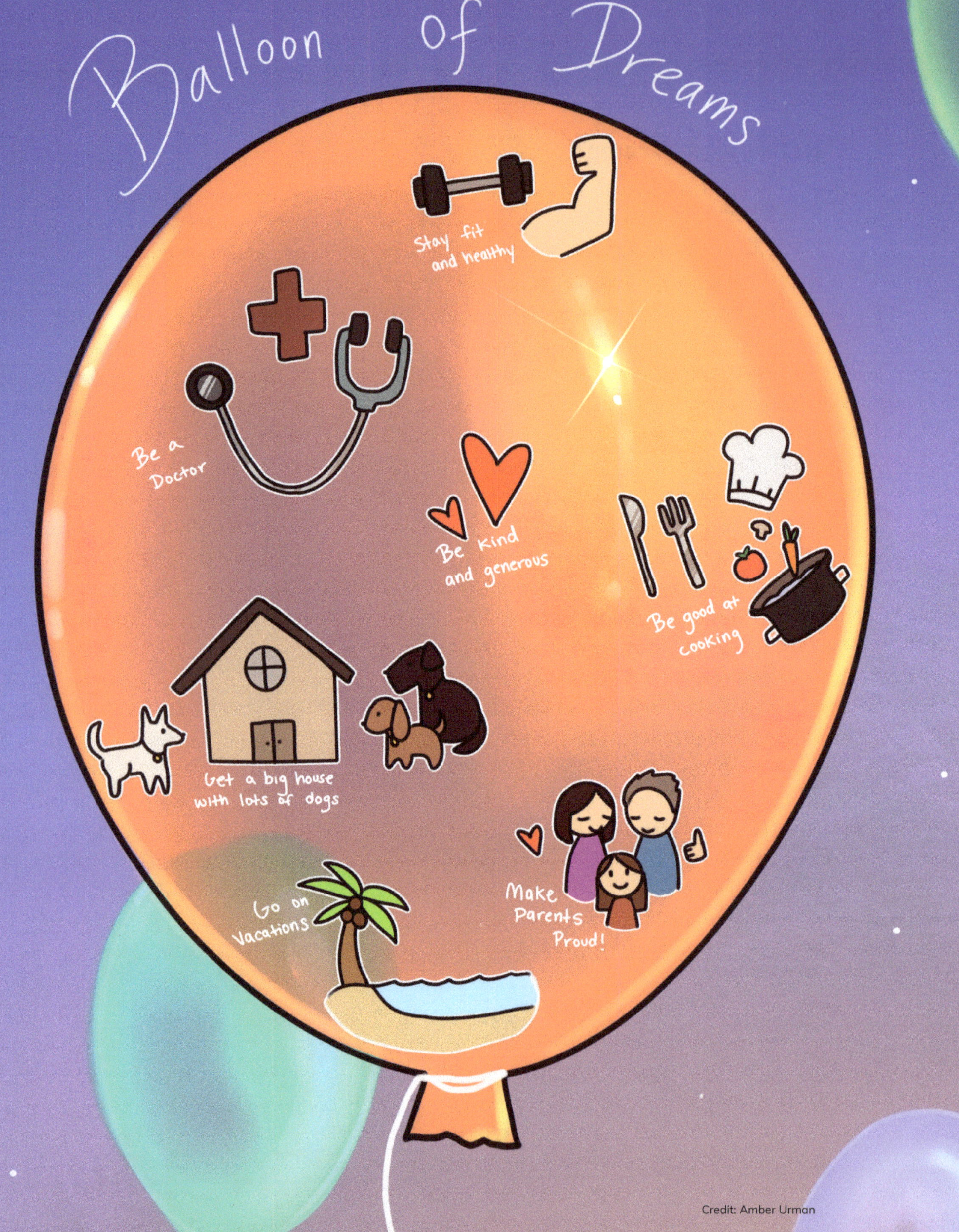

Credit: Amber Urman

Deflate & Re-inflate a Balloon

Find a real balloon and inflate it.

- Write down or draw something on the balloon that's been bothering you or a challenge you've faced.
- Then, carefully deflate the balloon.
- Take a moment to think about how it feels when the issue deflates. What changes?
- Now, reinflate the balloon and think about how it feels to see the issue come back.
- Share your experience with your friends, and discuss what you learned about coping with challenges. It's like experiencing the ups and downs of life through a balloon!

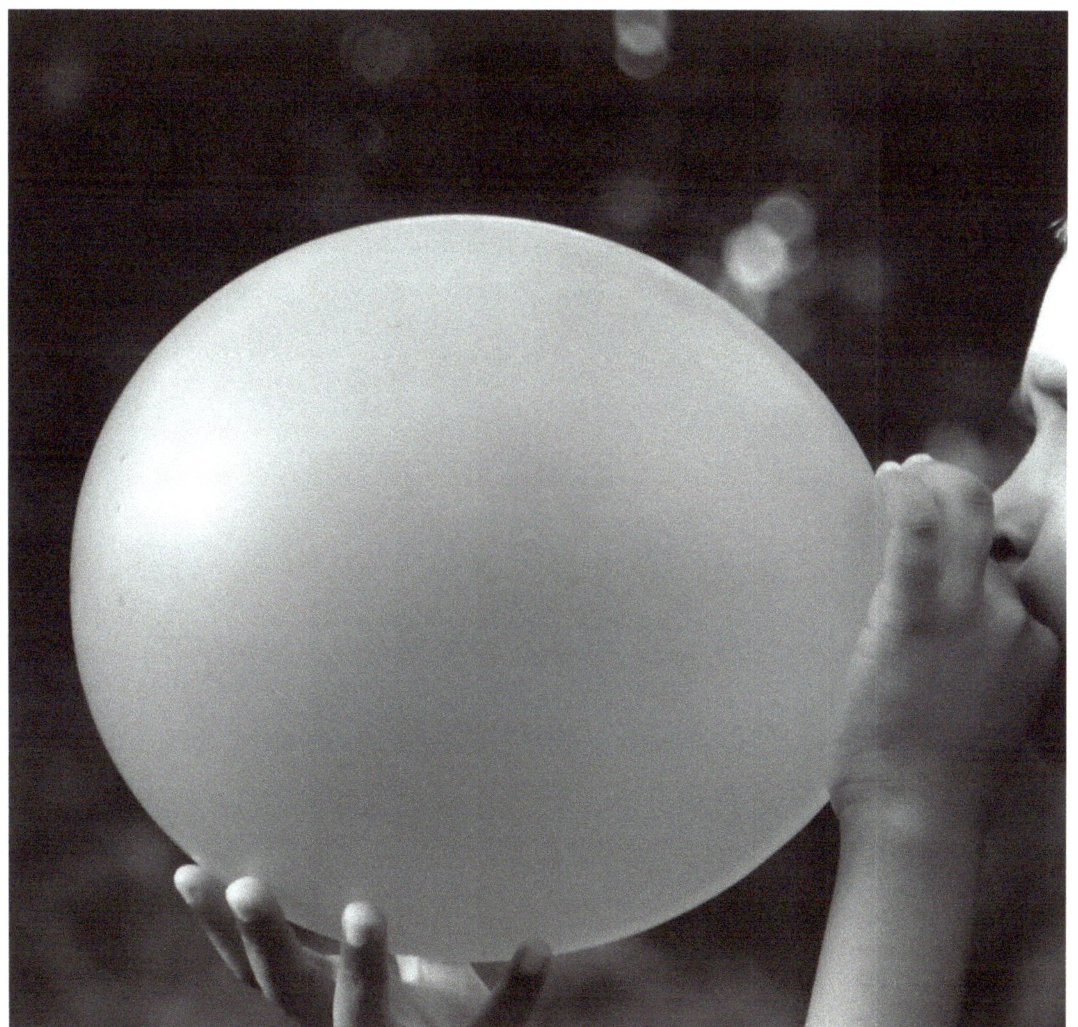

Design a Postcard You'll Never Send

Creating a "design a postcard you'll never send" in art therapy is a therapeutic way to express your thoughts and feelings. You imagine designing a postcard to send to someone, but you don't actually send it. It's like creating a personal message to vent, share your emotions, or say things you might not feel comfortable saying in real life.

This activity allows you to release bottled-up emotions, gain clarity, and explore your inner world through art. It creates a safe space to express yourself, providing a sense of relief and self-expression.

Use this free postcard template as a starting point.

POST CARD

Time-Travel Postcard

- Imagine you could travel to any time or place in history. Create a postcard from that era or location. Draw or paint a scene that represents what you'd see and experience there.
- Write a message on the back as if you're sending it to your friends from the past or future. Share your time-travel postcard with your friends and discuss the place you chose.

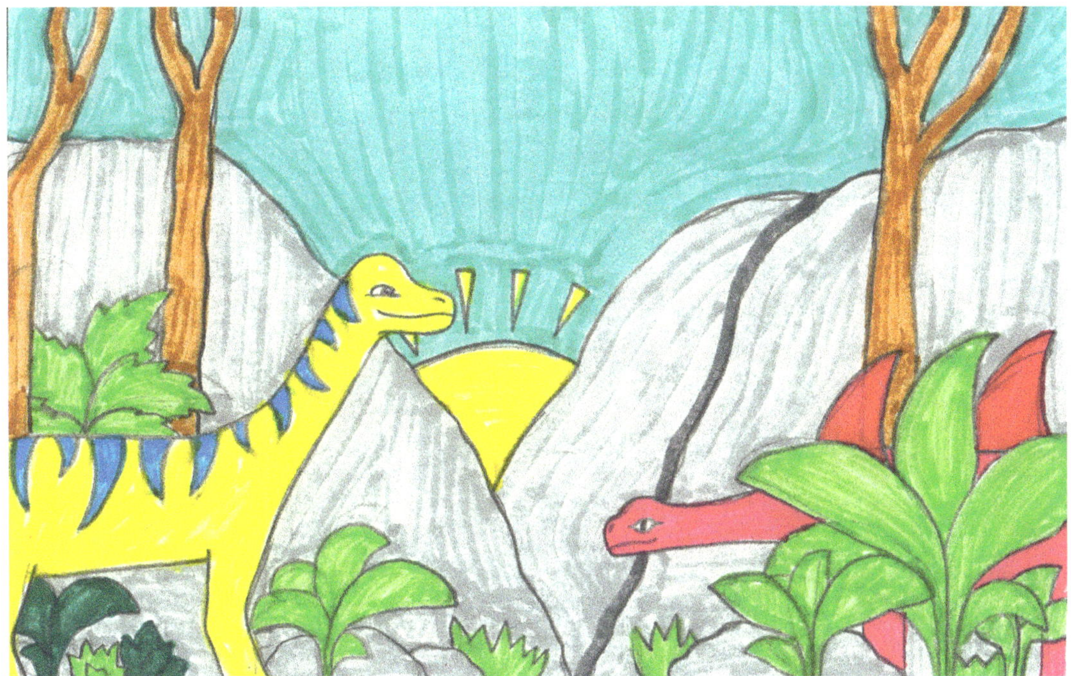

Credit: Ashley Yata

Emotional Landscape Postcard

- Choose an emotion or feeling you've experienced recently, like happiness, sadness, or excitement.
- Create a postcard that visually represents that emotion. Use colors, shapes, and images to convey how it feels.
- Write a message on the back that explains what the emotion means to you.
- Share your emotional landscape postcard with your friends and discuss how you each interpret and express emotions differently.

Hidden Talents Postcard

- Think about a talent or skill you have that you might not always share with others.
- Design a postcard that showcases that talent. Draw or paint something related to it. Write a message that briefly explains your talent and why you enjoy it.
- Share your hidden talents postcard with your friends, and maybe even inspire them to share their hidden talents too.

Fantasy World Postcard

- Think about your favorite book, movie, or fantasy world.
- Design a postcard featuring a scene or place from that world. Use your imagination to make it magical and exciting.
- Write a message as if you're sending it from that fantastical place to your friends in the real world.
- Share your fantasy world postcard and geek out with your friends about your favorite fictional worlds. It's like bringing your daydreams to life!

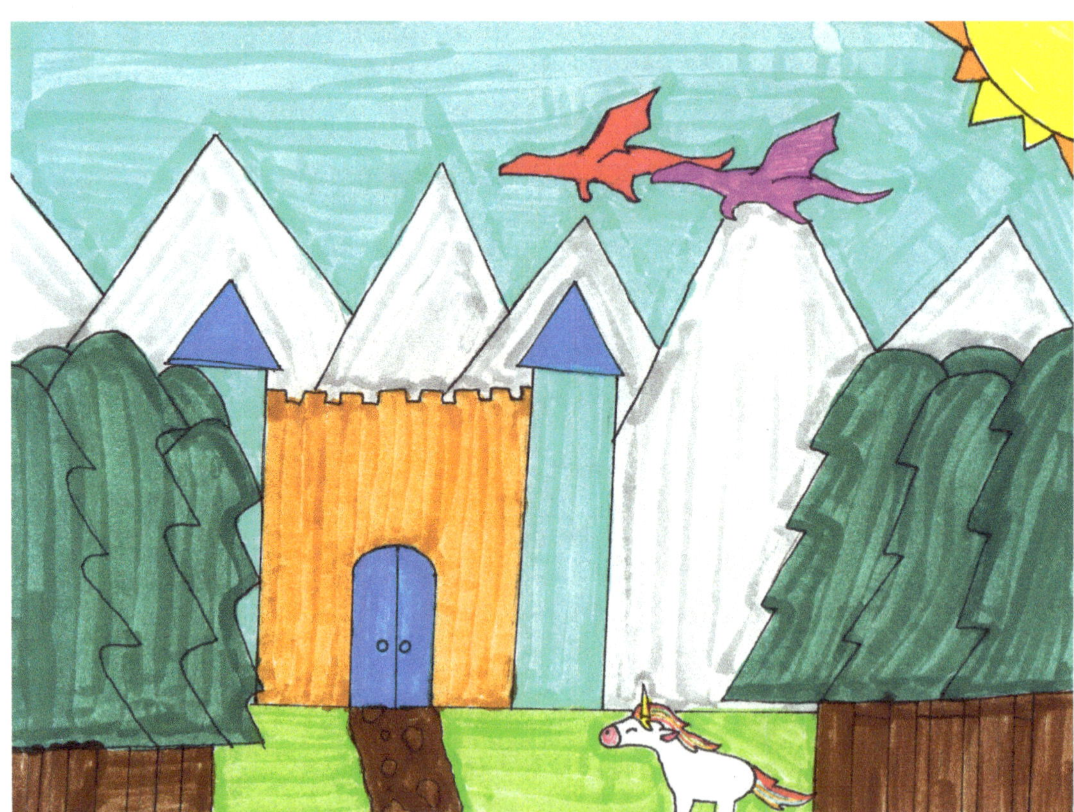

Credit: Ashley Yata

Dream Vacation Postcard

- Imagine your dream vacation destination.
- Create a postcard featuring that dream location. Draw the sights you'd love to see or activities you'd like to do.
- Write a message on the back as if you're sending it to your friends while on your dream trip.
- Share your dream vacation postcard with your friends and talk about your dream destinations and travel aspirations.

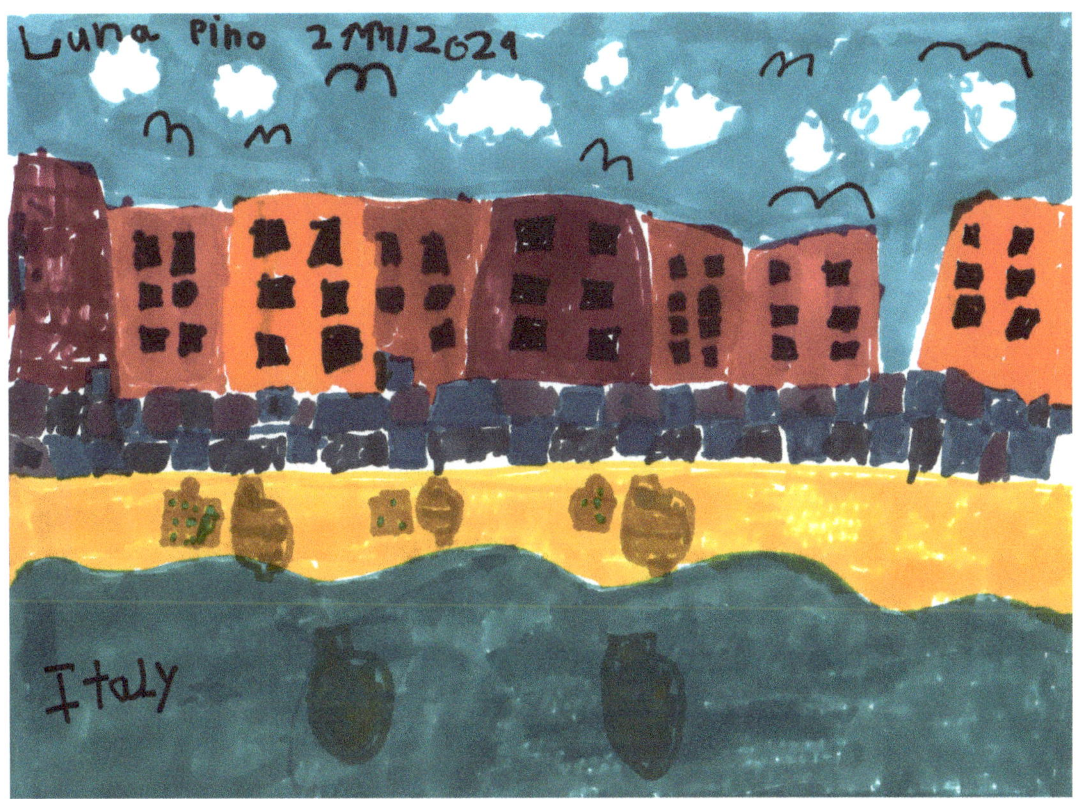

Credit: Luna Pino

Mental Health Resources

"Art speaks where words are unable to explain."

– Pam Holland

Art Therapy Resources

American Art Therapy Association: https://arttherapy.org/
Psychology.Org: https://www.psychology.org/resources/what-is-art-therapy/
Therapist Aid: https://www.therapistaid.com/search?query=art+therapy

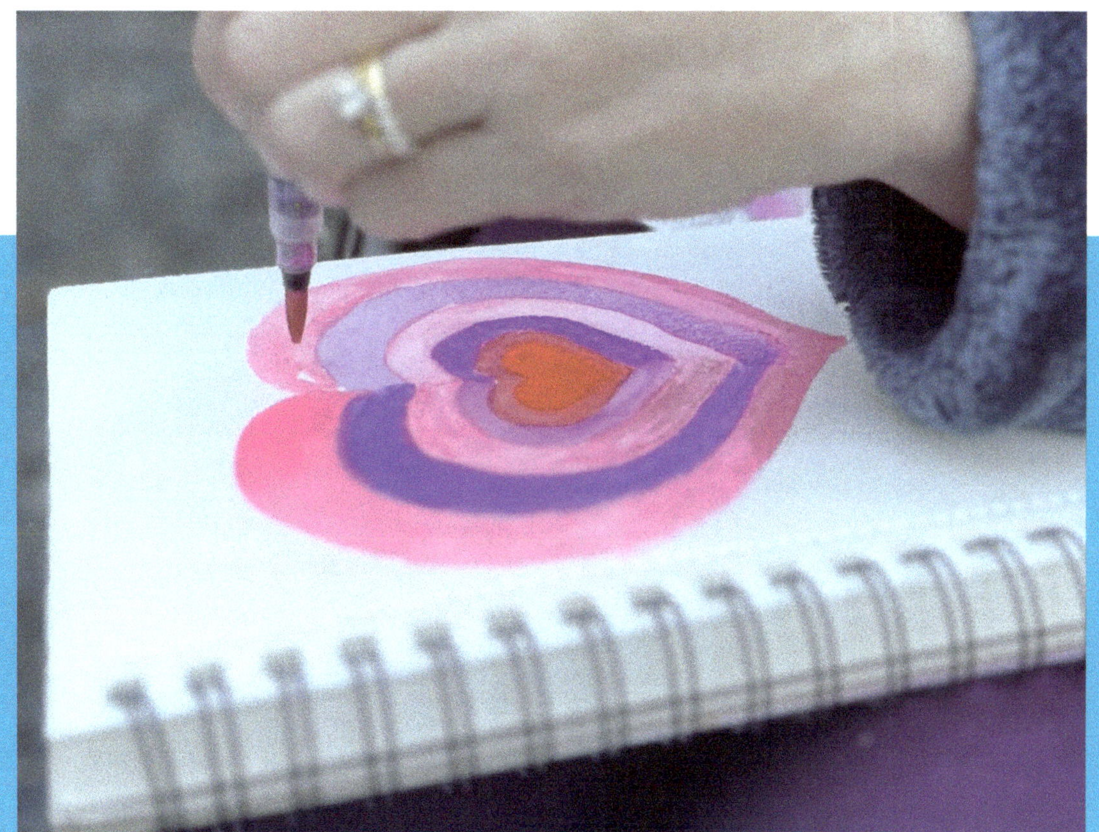

Crisis Support Resources

American Association of Poison Control Centers
1-800-222-1222

LGBT National Help Center
https://www.lgbthotline.org/
- LGBT National Hotline 1-888-843-4564
- LGBT National Youth Talkline
  1-800-246-7743
- LGBT National Senior Hotline
  1-888-234-7243
- LGBT National Coming Out Support
  Hotline 1-888-OUT-LGBT
  (888-688-5428)

Lifeline Crisis Lifeline (24/7)
https://988lifeline.org/
Call: 988
SMS: 988

National Council on Alcoholism and Drug Dependence Hope Line
https://ncadd.us/
1-800-662-4357

Emergency
911

National Suicide Prevention Line
- Toll-free at 1-800-273-TALK (8225)
- Text the Crisis Text Line (HELLO to 741741)
- Use the Lifeline Chat on the National Suicide Prevention Lifeline website

National Domestic Violence Hotline
1-800-799-SAFE (7233)
SMS: Text START to 88788

Self-Harm Crisis Text Line
https://www.crisistextline.org/
Text HOME to 741741

Local County Hotline Information (free and confidential)
- Contra Costa Crisis Center (925) 939-1916 or
Text 'HOPE' to 20121
- Crisis Support Services of Alameda County (800) 309-2131

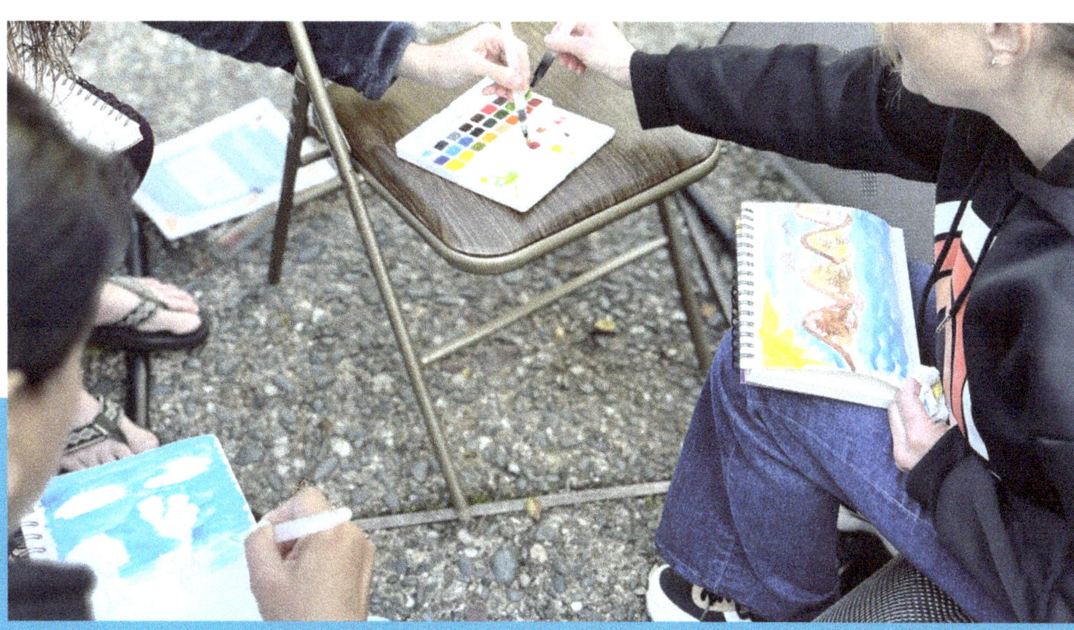

About the Author

Eme Williams is a 15-year old passionate creator, entrepreneur, and author of a mental health art therapy book debuting in April 2024. Currently, she is a high school sophomore aspiring to empower and inspire through entrepreneurship, service, and art therapy practices.

As Eme transitioned back to in-person school after the Covid-19 pandemic, she noticed how the pressures to perform and excel in academics, athletics, and extracurriculars have negatively impacted teens in her community. Through research, she became aware, and even more alarmed, that this local issue is just a fraction of a much larger global epidemic of adolescents struggling with anxiety and negative thoughts.

Under the guidance of her school counselor and mental health clinicians at the Discovering Counseling Center of the San Ramon Valley, she created a mental health art therapy book as a free resource for teens to learn how to manage their anxiety through mindfulness. "Therapy isn't about feeling better, it's about getting better at feeling." The mindfulness practice is executed through various art activities provided in the book, inspiring teens to learn how to "get better at feeling."

In April 2024, Eme plans to release her art therapy book on Amazon and donate hardcopies to local non-profit mental health organizations, such as the Discovery Counseling Center to promote her strong belief that everybody deserves access to all mental health resources needed, no matter their financial situation.